D1614045

Many Thanks to:

Jessie Amoss
for her modeling contributions
at age 86!

Terry Tucker, R.N.
for her continual inspiration
and friendship

and

Jugdeep Aggarwal
my husband, who supports me
in all my many projects

The Osteoporosis Exercise Book: Building Better Bones
Published by Osteo Physical Therapy
Copyright © 2008 by Sherri R. Betz, PT, GCS, CEEAA
ISBN 0967515203

The Osteoporosis Exercise Book:
Building Better Bones

Sherri R. Betz, PT
TheraPilates® Physical Therapy
    and Gyrotonic® Clinic
920-A 41st Avenue
Santa Cruz, CA 95062
831-476-3100
email: Sherri@TheraPilates.com

FOREWORD

As a physician who has established multiple osteoporosis programs over the past 15 years, I have accepted, almost as a matter of faith, that an active exercise program must be an integral part of any treatment plan which deals with the full scope of that disorder. For almost 10 years, women in my community- those with various degrees of osteopenia, osteoporosis, as well as those with and without osteoporotic fractures- have dutifully shown up for their twice-weekly exercise classes. I have always considered this remarkable although certainly not unique. I am sure that women all over this country join such programs believing that they will gain bone, develop strength and balance, prevent falls, and even prevent osteoporotic fractures- perhaps without the need to take any of those "harmful medications". But what is the real evidence that following the exercise program in this book (or any book) will be helpful to the sufferer with osteoporosis? Perhaps more important, how can the reader tell whether any given exercise program might actually be harmful, particularly if she or he doesn't have a degree in biomechanics or exercise physiology?

Over the past three years there have been more than 100 publications in the medical scientific literature dealing with the role of various types of exercise in the treatment of osteoporosis. Although a few of these reports are randomized controlled trials performed at University Centers—the highest form of scientific proof found in the medical literature—most are not. There has never been and probably never will be a controlled scientific study which demonstrates that exercise prevents osteoporotic fracture. Furthermore, my patients are not professional soccer players, teenage girls, middle-aged men or premenopausal women with normal bone mass. So what can we conclude from our medical scientific investigation? Decline in bone mineral density is a natural part of the aging process but can be highly modified and does not necessarily have to result in osteoporotic fracture. Various forms of exercise under different circumstances result in increased bone mass although there is no general agreement on the best form of exercise for everyone. This increase in bone mass may be maintained through exercise provided one exercises for life: even professional soccer players, it appears,

5

lose bone when they hang up their cleats. Finally, most hip fractures and many spine fractures are the result of falls. (No, I don't hold with that old adage, " I broke my hip and then I fell".) Any exercise regimen, which can train its adherents to develop better balance, should result in decreased fracture rates. It does appear that exercise programs such as the course outlined in this book can accomplish these objectives.

If you believe the medical scientific community is in the dark ages regarding exercise and osteoporosis, pick up any popular book on the subject at your local bookstore or supermarket. Notice the illustrations on the cover of one book picturing the instructor swinging the student (pronounced "V-I-C-T-I-M ") from the wrists (a good way to dislocate or even fracture your shoulder). Look at the pictures of exercises that put hundreds of pounds of mechanical stress on your lower back with crunches, lunges and recumbent leg thrusts against resistance. Note the maneuvers suggested which torque or twist the spine against resistance. Of course, as noted in one popular book, you could always build bone by taking up arm wrestling, preferably against a larger male opponent. Some of the books, notably Dr. Sydney Bonnick's book, do provide excellent general medical background on the subject of osteoporosis including solid information on nutrition and medication. Most however deal with popular myths such as the theory that stress decreases bone mass, toxic metals are the culprit, "weak" digestion causes osteoporosis, or that you must have the "18 nutrients essential for bones". Medical statistics suggest that around 35% of Caucasian women over age 50 will develop osteoporosis but if stress and inadequate boron stores could cause osteoporosis that figure would be closer to 95%. Many of these books also imply that you can simply do these exercises in the comfort of your own home after looking at the pictures (often diagrams of stick figure). Clearly what is needed is an osteoporosis exercise book written by a therapist, loaded with explicit photographs, which describe exercises which are not dangerous and can be performed by educated but not necessarily athletic postmenopausal women.

Not long ago, a patient of mine who had suffered multiple vertebral fractures brought me a copy of her church newspaper, which had her picture on the front page. She wanted to show me how well her recovery was progressing and how mobile and functional she had become with her exercise program.

The picture showed her on the top of a ladder with her back arched backwards and a paint roller in her hand painting the ceiling of the church. Outwardly I forced a smile but inside I was horrified. There is no book and no exercise program, which is a substitute for safety and common sense. In the pages that follow, however, I hope you will find illustrations of maneuvers which are safe, will increase your bone mass and that you can follow for life.

David R. Gelbart, M.D.
Medical Director
Osteoporosis Diagnostic Centers
A Member of the Osteoporosis Care Centers Network

8

INTRODUCTION

Osteoporosis has become a national epidemic. Osteoporosis is the gradual and silent loss of bone, primarily affecting post-menopausal Caucasian women. Statistics show that 1 in every 2 post-menopausal women will be affected by osteoporosis. In my practice as a physical therapist I have found that the patients I work with are younger and younger. I used to only treat osteoporosis in nursing homes and now I see patients with bone loss more frequently in outpatient facilities. It has been reported that 20 million Americans are affected by osteoporosis and this number is expected to rise to 53 million by the year 2030. What are we doing wrong? In my opinion, the American lifestyle is the culprit. We base our habits of daily living on convenience and time management. We have computers for shopping, TV to entertain us, washing machines, elevators, escalators, cars and high tech devices to "save time" and to make our lives more efficient. These high tech efficiencies are killing us!

What can we do to help ourselves? Although nutrition is not the focus of this book, I have included charts with permission from Christiane Northrup, MD, full of calcium-rich foods to include in the diet. Nutrition, environment, healthy relationships and exercise are all part of a balanced lifestyle in which all of the components must be included to stay healthy, build bone and prevent as well as reverse osteoporosis. It has been shown that exercise alone can halt the progression of osteoporosis in most cases. I have seen patients gain from 6-15% bone density in one year through the recommended program that follows.

Osteoporosis most commonly affects the spinal vertebrae, hips and wrists. Post-menopausal women have a greater susceptibility to bone loss due to the decrease of estrogen and progesterone. These hormones work together to stimulate bone and inhibit bone loss. This is the reason many women are placed on HRT (hormone replacement therapy) after menopause. The risks of HRT are well known and many women are opting to go the "natural route" through lifestyle modification, nutritional changes and exercise.

My goal as a physical therapist is to dispel the myth that aging means decline and that arthritis and osteoporosis (resulting in bones that are exceptionally brittle) are a natural part of aging.

In underdeveloped countries where the calcium intake is much lower tha America, 80-year-old women are seen in a full squat waiting for the bus. Japan, women don't get breast cancer and osteoporosis at anywhere nea the rate that Americans do. *(Campbell 2005)* Their diet is low in fat, low in re meat, and high in calcium and soy. They get their calcium from greens, se vegetables, fish and soy. By making small changes gradually you can rea the benefits of renewed health, vitality and stronger bones!

The number one reason that people are admitted as nursing home residen is due to hip fractures which cause them to lose the ability to ambula (walk).

Some of the risk factors for Osteoporosis are:
- nulliparity (never having children)
- history of glucocorticoid (cortisone) therapy
- premature or early surgical menopause (before age 40)
- heavy alcohol consumption
- family history
- Caucasian female- slight build, fair skin, blonde
- smoking
- hypothyroidism
- sedentary lifestyle
- high fat/high protein diet
- medications which sedate or alter balance increase risk of fractures in elderly 2-3 times

BONE DENSITY TESTING (DEXA)

To find out how your bones are doing you can have a bone density te done. DEXA (Dual Energy X-ray Absorptiometry) is the state of the art bor screening tool. The cost is relatively low and is covered by most heal insurances. It is very safe with little exposure to radiation. The technicia can even stay in the same room with you without protection because th radiation is so low. It is recommended to get a baseline at age of 40 ar every 2 years thereafter to check for bone loss.

IF YOU HAVE A FRACTURE:

IF YOU HAVE A FRACTURE you should consult a physical therapist experienced in treating osteoporosis to supervise your program.   The BEGINNER EXERCISES would be appropriate for someone with a fracture or a recent fracture.

If you are interested in a program for prevention start with the BEGINNER PROGRAM and when you can complete all the exercises easily and without discomfort start the INTERMEDIATE EXERCISES.   Always begin with a warm-up activity like walking, marching in place, or gentle tai chi maneuvers so that your muscles will be warm and protected from strains.

IMPORTANT POINTS FOR FRACTURE PREVENTION:

1.   Do not forward bend or round your spine in sitting or standing especially when lifting heavy objects or lifting objects from the floor! This puts too much pressure on the vertebral bodies (front of the spine) and places the vertebrae at risk for fracture.

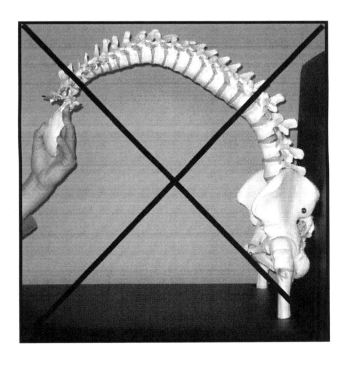
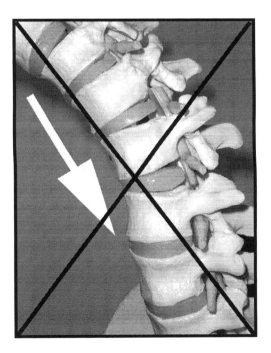

2. Do not side bend, twist or rotate your spine in sitting or standi

positions!

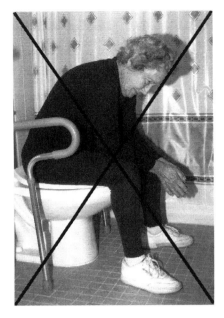

3. Do not perform the pigeon pose from Yoga (too much force come down through the hip joint with the hip in a rotated position)!!

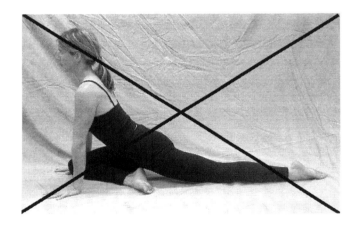

HOW TO BEGIN YOUR EXERCISE PROGRAM:

1. Always get your yearly physical before beginning any exercise progran Get your physician's clearance (bring this book with you to yo appointment) before beginning any exercise program.

2. If you have chest pain, feel faint, nausea, dizziness, heart racing palpitations STOP exercising and call your physician.

IF YOU HAVE A FRACTURE:

IF YOU HAVE A FRACTURE you should consult a physical therapist experienced in treating osteoporosis to supervise your program. The BEGINNER EXERCISES would be appropriate for someone with a fracture or a recent fracture.

If you are interested in a program for prevention start with the BEGINNER PROGRAM and when you can complete all the exercises easily and without discomfort start the INTERMEDIATE EXERCISES. Always begin with a warm-up activity like walking, marching in place, or gentle tai chi maneuvers so that your muscles will be warm and protected from strains.

IMPORTANT POINTS FOR FRACTURE PREVENTION:

1. Do not forward bend or round your spine in sitting or standing especially when lifting heavy objects or lifting objects from the floor! This puts too much pressure on the vertebral bodies (front of the spine) and places the vertebrae at risk for fracture.

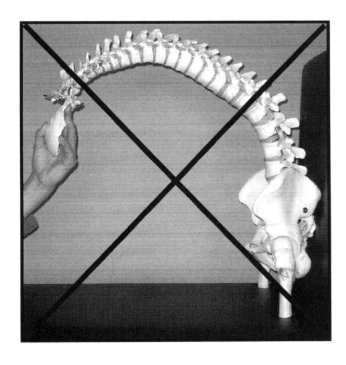
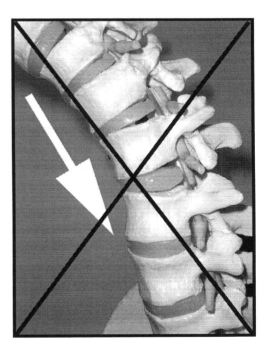

2. Do not side bend, twist or rotate your spine in sitting or standing positions!

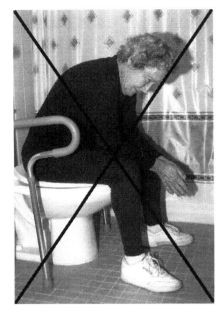

3. Do not perform the pigeon pose from Yoga (too much force comes down through the hip joint with the hip in a rotated position)!!

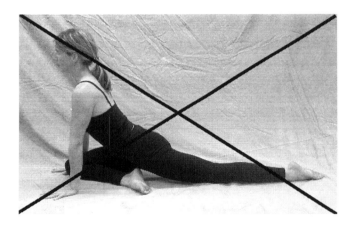

HOW TO BEGIN YOUR EXERCISE PROGRAM:

1. Always get your yearly physical before beginning any exercise program. Get your physician's clearance (bring this book with you to your appointment) before beginning any exercise program.

2. If you have chest pain, feel faint, nausea, dizziness, heart racing palpitations STOP exercising and call your physician.

3. If you have pain with any exercise STOP. Attempt to modify the exercise by making the movement smaller or less intense. If you cannot tolerate the exercise without pain, STOP altogether and consult your physician. You might ask the physician for a physical therapy prescription so that you can get a supervised program designed for your needs.

4. Perform all exercises slowly and gently. Don't push to exhaustion.

5. You should start with 5-10 repetitions of each exercise then increase to 15 repetitions at a rate of adding 5 repetitions per week. When you can perform 15 repetitions easily you can begin to add weights to your ankles and use dumbbells in your hands. If you don't want to purchase fancy equipment use 12 or 16 oz. sport bottles of water for dumbbells and tie 1 lb. rice bags around your ankles.

6. When you can easily perform all of the INTERMEDIATE level exercises 15 times each you can begin the ADVANCED EXERCISES using the same method as described in #3.

7. Begin doing the exercises every day preferably at the same time of day and when your strength has improved then you can decrease the exercises to every other day.

8. Begin a walking program along with the exercises. Start by walking 5 minutes away from your home, mark the spot and turn around and walk back home. Do this for one week. The 2nd week walk 7-8 minutes away from your home, mark the spot, turn around and walk back home. The 3rd week walk 10 minutes away from your home, mark the spot, turn around and walk back home. The 4th week walk 12-13 minutes away from your home, mark the spot, turn around and walk back home. The 5th week walk 15 minutes away from your home, mark the spot, turn around and walk back home. So, by the 5th week you will have achieved your goal of a 30-minute walk every day. To progress with your walking program, try to walk farther which means you'll be walking faster. Don't try to walk more that 30 minutes so that you limit your exercise time and help you fit your walk easily into your daily schedule. If you want to increase the intensity of your walk, try a hilly terrain, a park or trail. I recommend walking in a beautiful place where you can get lots of fresh air and stimulation from the environment. Also getting a partner to walk with you helps with motivation!

FOODS CONTAINING HIGH LEVELS OF CALCIUM

Green Leafy Vegetables (1 cup cooked unless specified):
- collard greens   300 mg.
- wild greens (lamb's quarters, wild onions)   350
- broccoli   150
- kale   179
- spinach   278
- turnip greens   229
- beet greens   165
- bok choy   200
- mustard greens   150
- rhubarb   348
- watercress (raw)   53
- parsley (raw)   122
- dandelion greens   147

Sea Vegetables (1 cup)
- hijiki   610
- wakame   520
- kombu   305
- agar-agar (dry flakes)   400
    (Kanten Flakes- 16 tablespoons
        used as a thickener for sauces, etc.
- dulse (dry)   567

Fish (bones: the major source of calcium in fish)
- sardines 3.5 oz. Can-drained with bones   300
- salmon (canned)   431
- oysters (raw)   226

Beans and Legumes
- tofu-firm 4 oz.   80-150
- tempeh 4 oz.   172
- garbanzo beans (chickpeas) 1 cup   150
- black beans 1 cup   135
- pinto beans 1cup   128
- corn tortilla   60

Nuts and Seeds
- ground sesame seeds (Tahini) 3 tablespoons   300
- almonds   1 cup   300
- sunflower seeds 1 cup (hulled)   174
- brazil nuts 1 cup   260
- hazelnuts 1 cup   282

Other Sources
- blackstrap molasses 1 T   137
- orange juice- calcium fortified-Minute Maid   210

Mineral Waters - 1 liter
- Perrier   140
- Mendocino   380
- San Pellegrino   200
- Apollinaris   91
- Contexeville   451

Dairy
- skim milk 1 cup   300
- nonfat yogurt 1 cup   294
- low fat cottage cheese 1 cup   150

Herbs (mineral-rich dark green leafy vegetables)
- Yellow dock leaves/roots
- Dandelion leaves/roots
- Plantain leaves
- Nettle leaves
- Raspberry leaves/canes/berries
- Mugwort leaves
- Comfrey leaves/flower stalks
- Red Clover blossoms
- Clean eggshells/bones

Food Chart is printed with permission from Dr. Christiane Northrup's Women's Bodies, Women's Wisdom text.

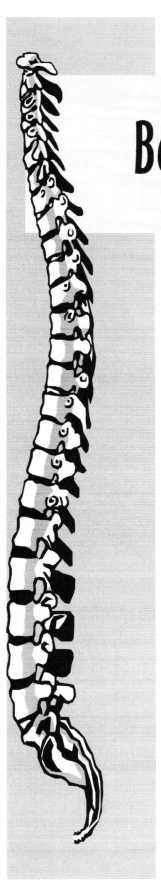

Beginner Level Exercises

SLUMPED SITTING POSTURE

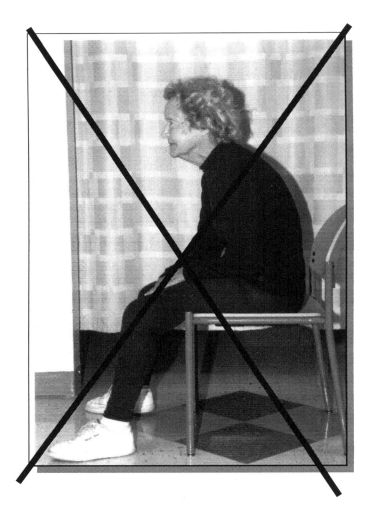 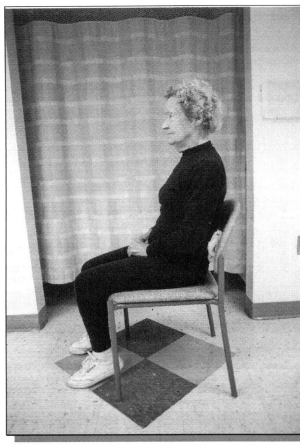

Avoid slumped sitting. Do not sit in chairs without your back fully supported. Use a pillow or towel roll to support your lumbar spine (low back) if necessary. Slumping makes the osteoporosis curve in the back worse and can cause further damage to the vertebrae.

18

TRUNK EXTENSION IN SITTING

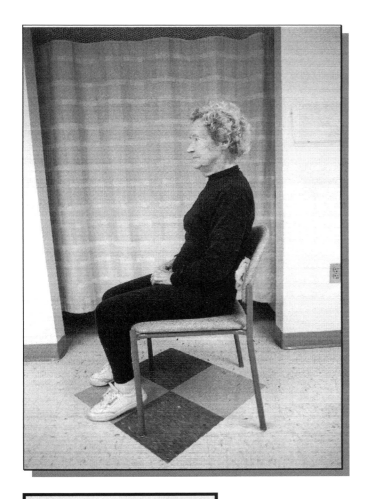

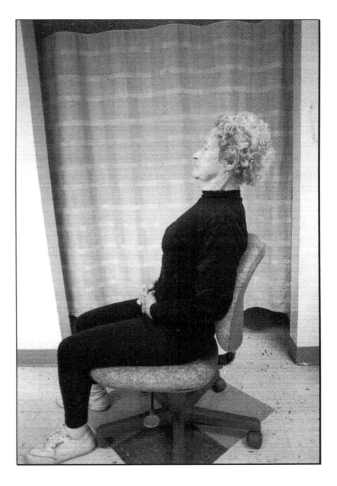

Sit all the way back in a straight back standard chair or desk chair. Place a towel roll behind the small of your back. Inhale and press your shoulder blades into the chair back. Hold 5 seconds. Exhale. Repeat 10 times. *Optional Stretch: Hands behind head, lift breastbone up.*

19

SITTING ARM RAISES

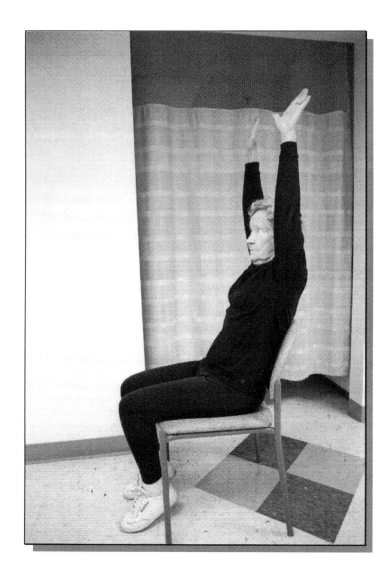

Sit all the way back in a chair. Lean backwards and let the chair fully suppo[rt] your back. Keep your feet on the floor. Inhale, and as you exhale raise you[r] arms straight upwards and reach for the ceiling. Keep your shoulder blades down. Hold 5 seconds. Repeat 10 times.

20

HIP HINGE IN SITTING

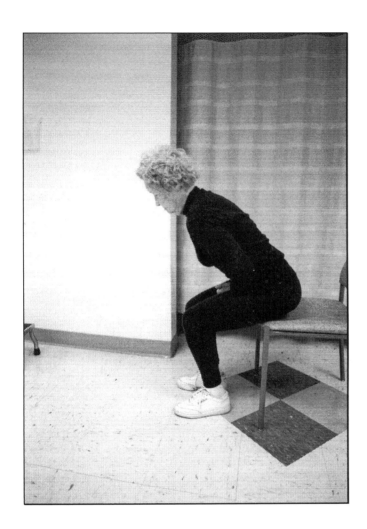 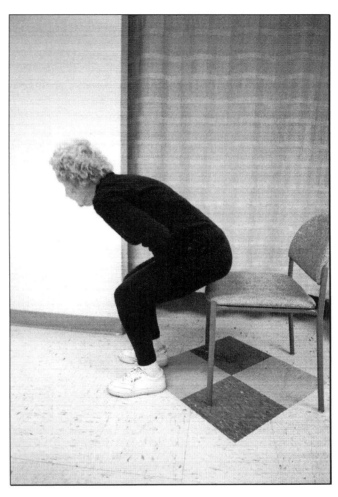

Scoot to the front of a chair. Adjust your feet behind your knees. Keep your feet pointed straight ahead and your knees apart. Bend at the <u>hips</u> to lean forward. If you place you hands on the tops of your thighs where the crease is you will be at your hip line. This is where you should bend instead of rounding the spine. Come up to a full standing position and sit back down slowly being sure to bend at the hips. Repeat 10 times. Try always to get out of chairs this way without using your hands. This will also help to strengthen your legs.

21

"T" EXERCISE SITTING

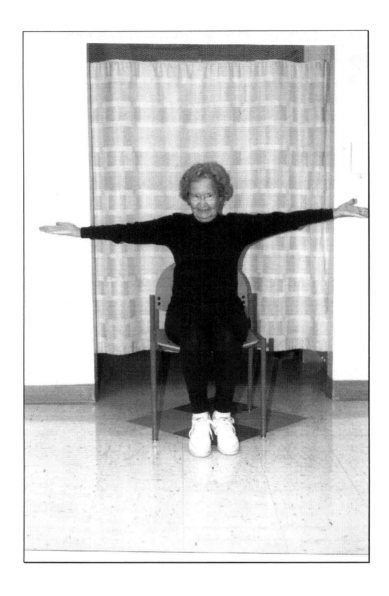

Sit in a chair. Hold your hands out in front of you with palms upward. Inhale and as you exhale open your arms as far as you can with elbows straight. Draw the shoulder blades together. Hold 5 seconds and repeat 10 times.

22

SITTING KNEE EXTENSIONS

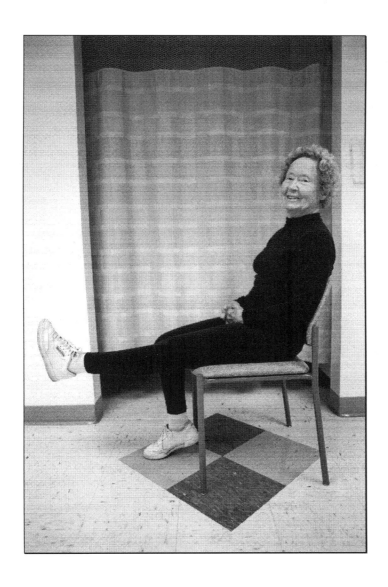

Sit all the way back in a chair. Lean backwards and let the chair fully support your back. Raise your foot upwards until your knee is fully straight. Tighten the muscle above your kneecap. Hold 5 seconds. Repeat 10 times.

CHAIR RISES

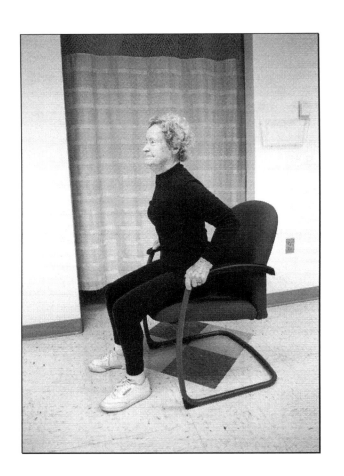 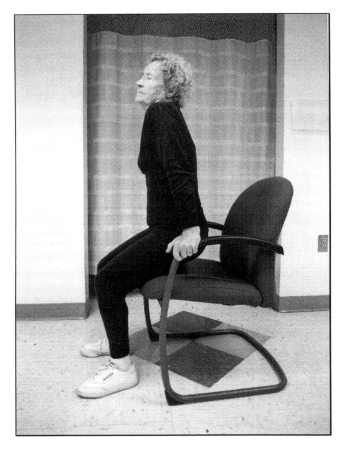

Sit at the edge of a chair with armrests. Inhale, and as you exhale press the breastbone upward. Try to straighten your arms.   Press your armpits downward. Hold 5 seconds and repeat 10 times.

24

HIP FLEXOR (PSOAS) STRETCH

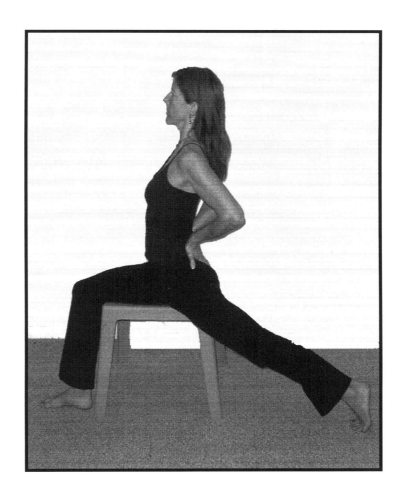

Sit at the edge of a chair without armrests or turn to the side in a chair with armrests. Place your hands on the back of your pelvis and press your sacrum (tailbone) down. Lift the pubic bone upwards. Extend one leg back behind you keeping your heel aimed at the ceiling. Breathe deeply as your hold the stretch for 30 seconds feeling a stretch in the front of the hip and groin of the leg that is extended back.

25

RESTING POSITION

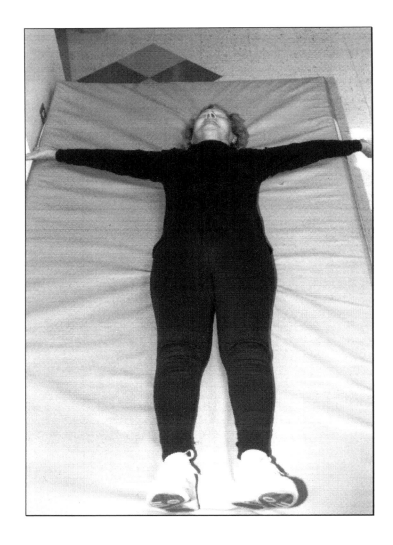

Lie flat on your back with arms extended out and hands palm up.
This will help to reverse the curve in your spine. Hold 3 minutes. Practice
deep breathing allowing your belly to expand as you inhale.

26

PELVIC TILT

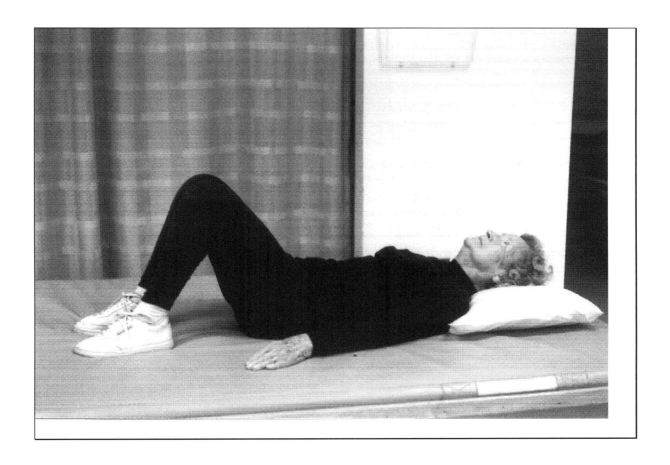

Lie on your back. Tighten your buttocks. Inhale, and as you exhale bring your hip bones toward your rib cage. Press your back into the floor and hold for 5 seconds. Inhale and repeat 10 times.

BRIDGE UP

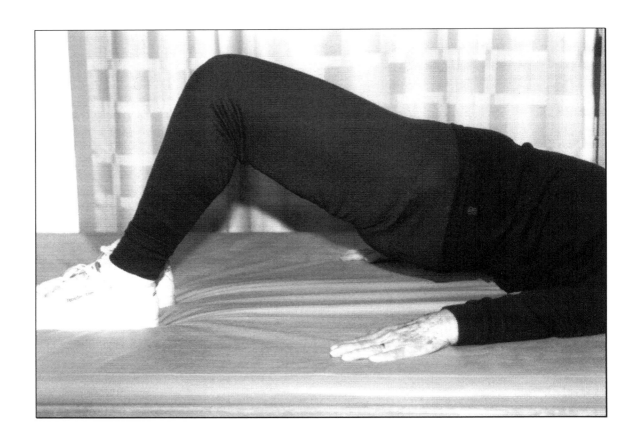

Lie on your back. Inhale, and as you exhale lift buttocks up off the floor and
peel the spine up one vertebra at a time. Stop when you are standing
between your shoulder blades. Avoid going up to the neck. Hold 5 seconds.
Inhale, and as you exhale roll down one bone at a time. Repeat 10 times.

28

PRONE: 2 PILLOWS

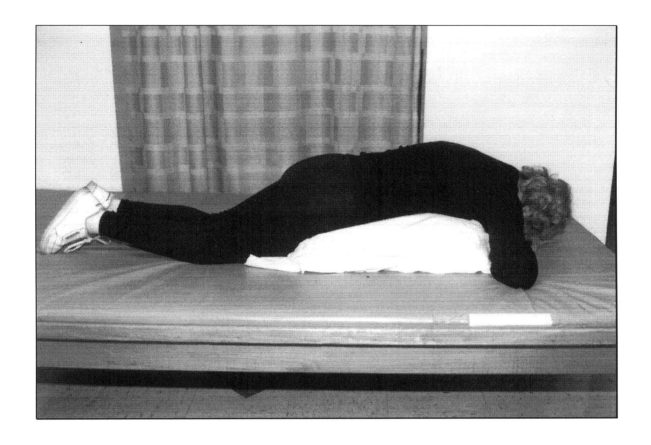

If you cannot lie flat on your stomach try propping 2 large pillows under your chest. Rest here for a few minutes each day.

29

PRONE: 1 PILLOW

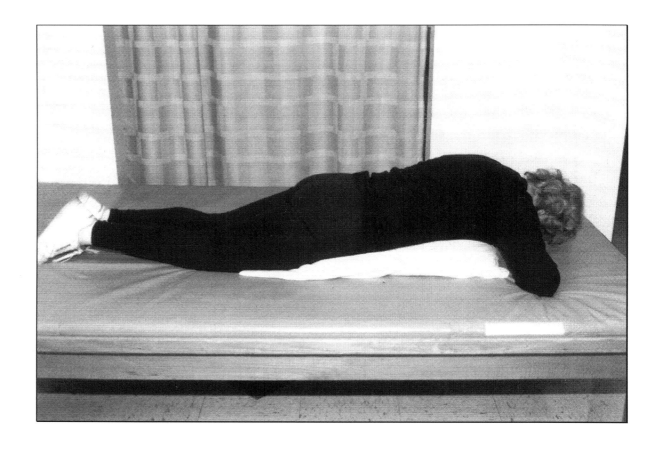

As you progress, begin to take out pillows. Rest here for a few minutes eac
day.

30

PRONE

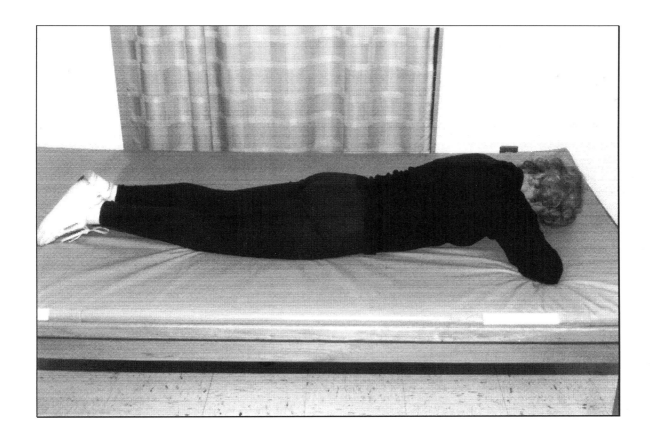

Progress to resting on your stomach with your hands stacked under your forehead to support your neck for a few minutes each day. Practice deep breathing into your belly.

31

PRONE ON ELBOWS

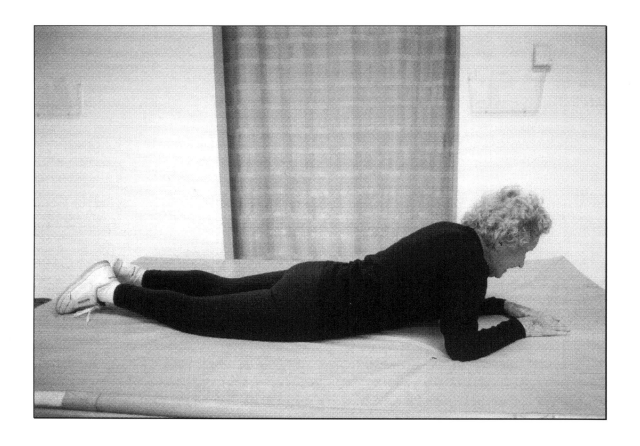

Rest on your elbows for a few minutes each day. Keep your shoulders dow
and keep trying to lift your breastbone.

32

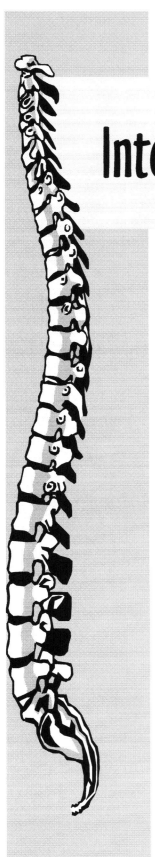

Intermediate Level Exercises

SINGLE KNEE TO CHEST

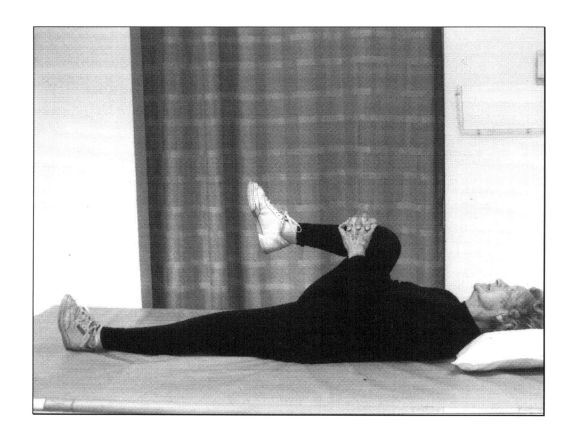

Lie on your back. Bring your knee toward your chest. Avoid pressure on the ribcage. Hold 30 seconds. Repeat on each leg.

37

PIRIFORMIS (HIP) STRETCH

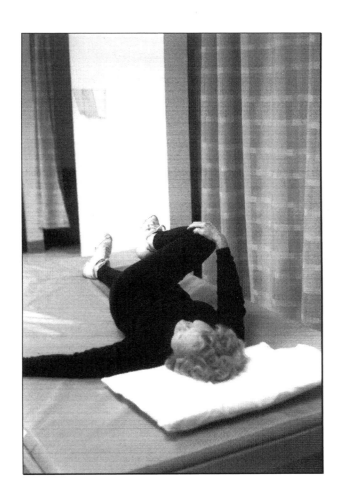 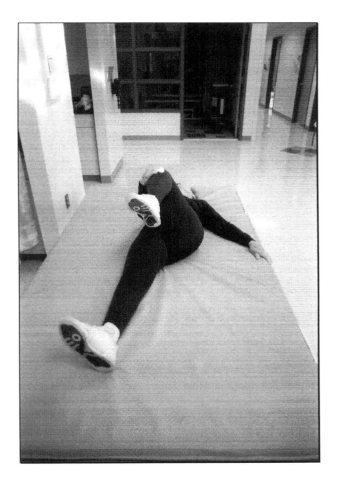

Lie on your back. Bring your left knee towards your chest. Grab the left shin with the right hand and pull across until you feel a stretch in the left outer hip area. Keep the left hip down. Hold 30 seconds. Repeat on each leg.

35

CROSSED LEG STRETCH

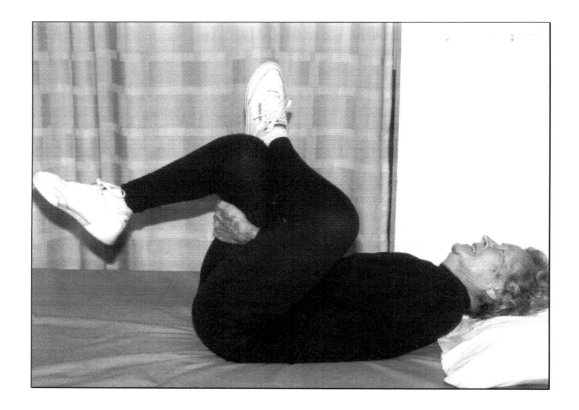

Lie on your back. Place your left shin on your right thigh. Using both hands gently draw your right thigh towards you until you feel a stretch in the left buttock. Keep your shoulder blades on the mat. Hold 30 seconds and repeat on each leg.

HAMSTRING STRETCH

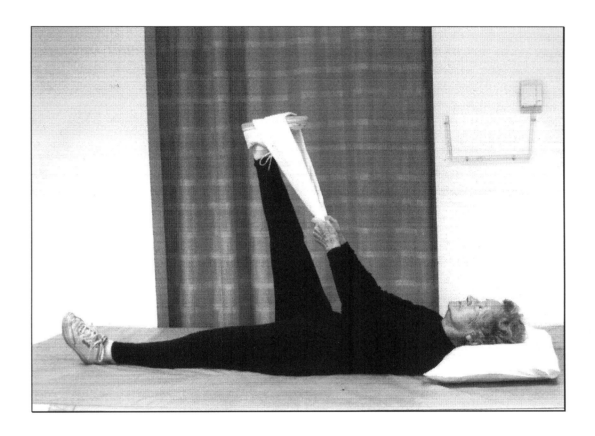

Lie on your back. Bend your right knee toward your chest and place a strap or towel around the arch of your right foot. Extend your right knee until it is straight and aim your foot toward the ceiling. You should feel a stretch behind your knee. Keep your shoulder blades on the mat. Hold 30 seconds and repeat on each leg.

1 LEG BRIDGE

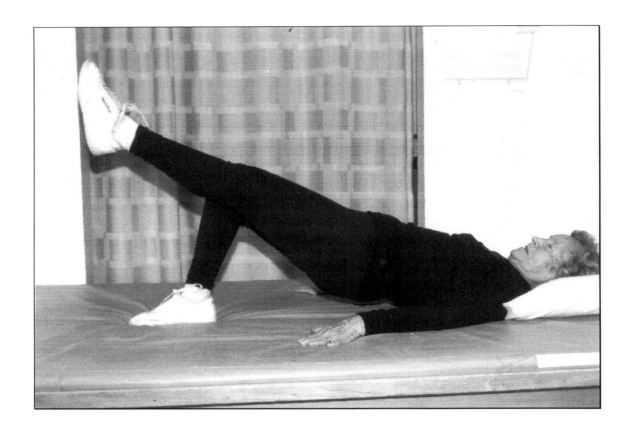

Lie on your back. Extend one leg and keep the knees together. Inhale and
then exhale as you peel the spine off the mat until you are standing betwee
the shoulder blades. Lift buttocks up off the floor. Keep the pelvis level.
Hold 5 seconds. Exhale to lower down. If too difficult just bend the top kne
and march in place. Repeat 10 times.

38

ABDOMINAL & HIP STRENGTHENING EXERCISE

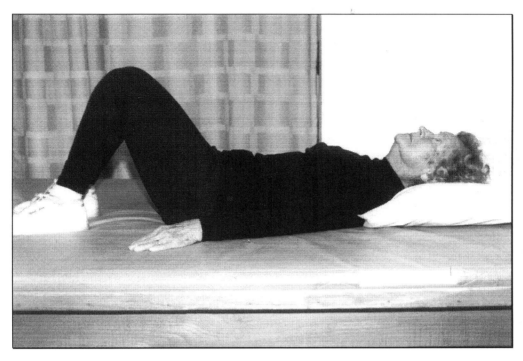

Lie on your back with knees bent.

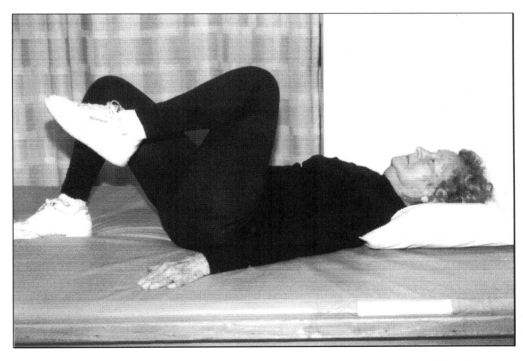

Inhale as you bring one knee towards your chest.

39

ABDOMINAL & HIP EXERCISE CONTINUED

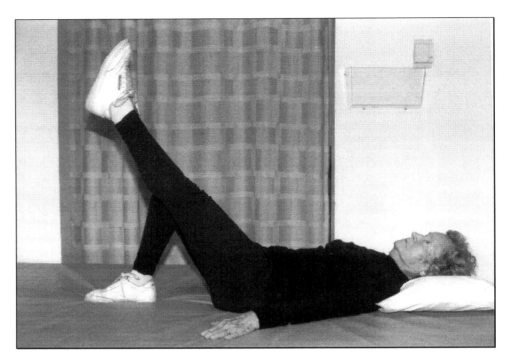

Keeping the low back flat, exhale and extend the knee until the leg is straig
and slowly lower it down.

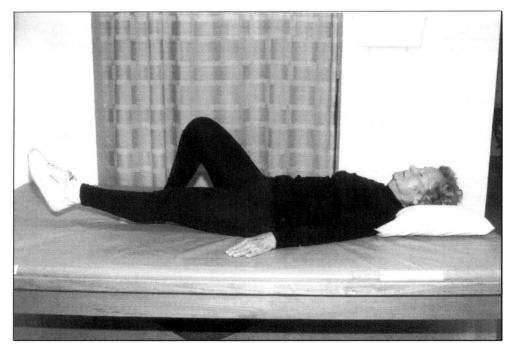

Touch the heel to the floor and repeat the sequence. Repeat 10 times on
each leg.

PRESS UP

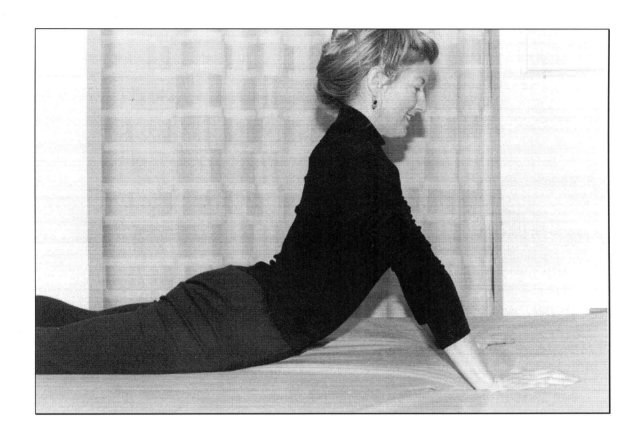

Place your hands underneath your shoulders. Inhale, and as you exhale, push up using only your arms. Keep your stomach drawn in and send your tailbone towards your feet. Keep your shoulder blades down and back. Try to straighten your elbows. Do not hold. Go up and down slowly. Repeat 10 times.

41

SINGLE ARM RAISES

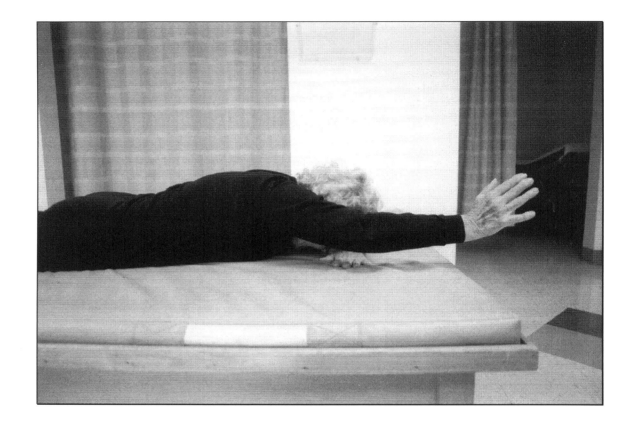

Place your left hand under your forehead with the palm down. Reach your right arm straight out with thumb up. Inhale, and as you exhale draw your shoulder blade down and raise your arm up 2-3" off the floor. Repeat 10 times. Repeat with opposite arm.

PRONE HIP EXTENSION

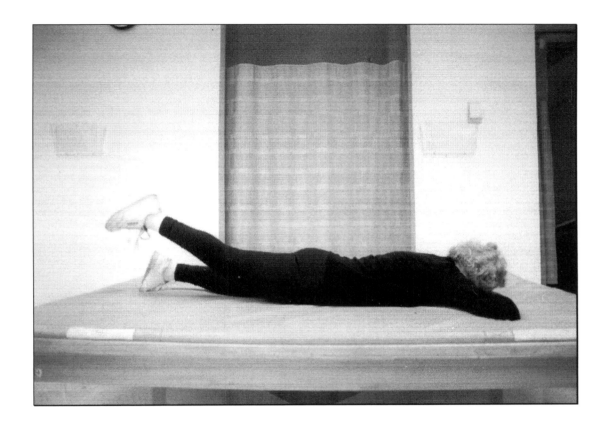

Lie on your stomach with both hands palms down under your forehead. Keep your pelvis and pubic bone connected to the mat. Inhale, and as you exhale, lift one leg with the knee straight. Hold 5 seconds and repeat 10 times.

PRONE OPPOSITE ARM & LEG RAISE

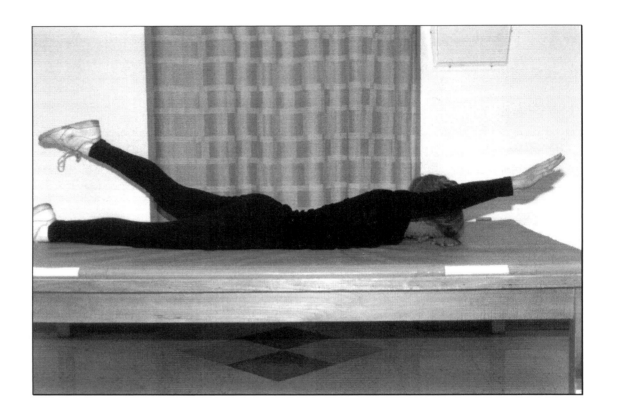

Lie on your stomach with the left hand palm down under your forehead. Inhale, and as you exhale, raise the right arm and left leg up. Keep the elbow and the knee straight. Hold 5 seconds and repeat 10 times.

44

PRONE BILATERAL ARM RAISES

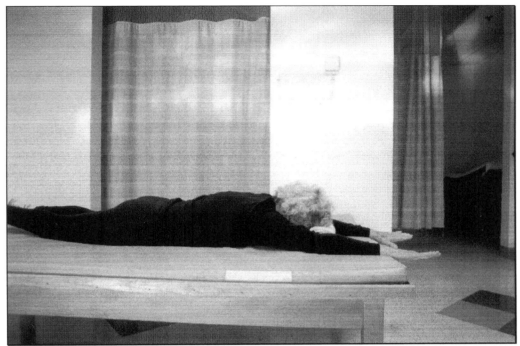

Start with a towel roll under your forehead.

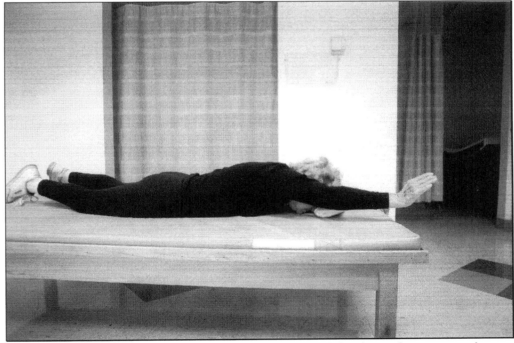

Inhale and as you exhale, draw your shoulder blades down and reach both arms straight out and lift them 2-3" with elbows straight. Hold 5 seconds and repeat 10 times.

45

MODIFIED PRONE BILATERAL ARM RAISE

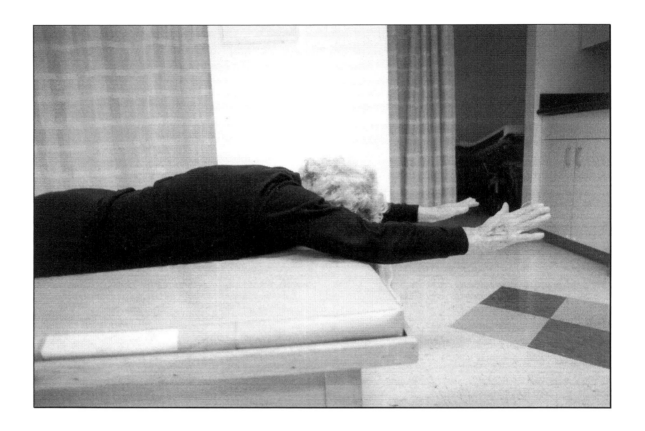

Lie on your stomach with your head at the edge of the bed and a towel roll under your forehead. Inhale, and as you exhale, draw your shoulder blades down and extend your arms off the edge of the bed. Lift your arms 2-3" with the elbows straight. Hold 5 seconds and repeat 10 times.

46

"W" EXERCISE

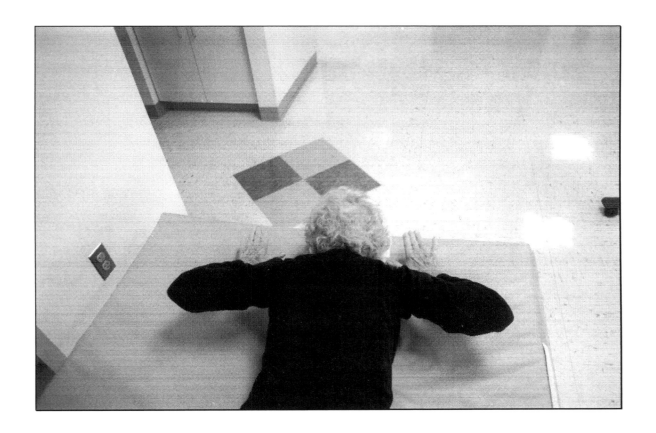

Lie on your stomach with a towel roll under your forehead. Place your hands by your ears. Lift both your hands and your elbows up. Draw your shoulder blades together and down. Hold 5 seconds and repeat 10 times.

47

HIP HINGE IN STANDING

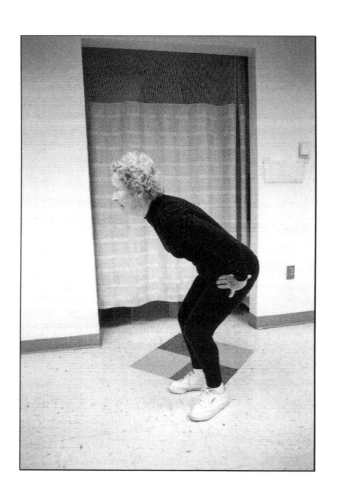 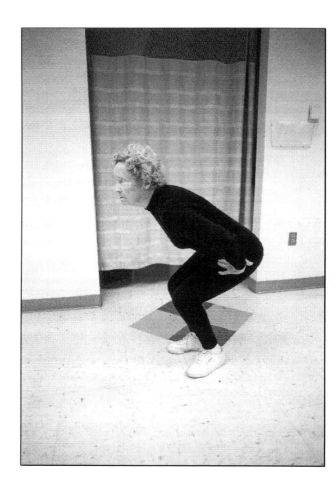

Place your hand in the crease underneath your abdomen. This is the area where your hip joint is located. (Usually at your underwear line) Bend at the <u>hips</u> to lean forward. Keep your tailbone lifted and your chest up. Keep feet pointed straight ahead and knees apart. When bending forward for daily tasks always bend at the hip <u>instead</u> of rounding the spine.

48

HAMSTRING STRETCH

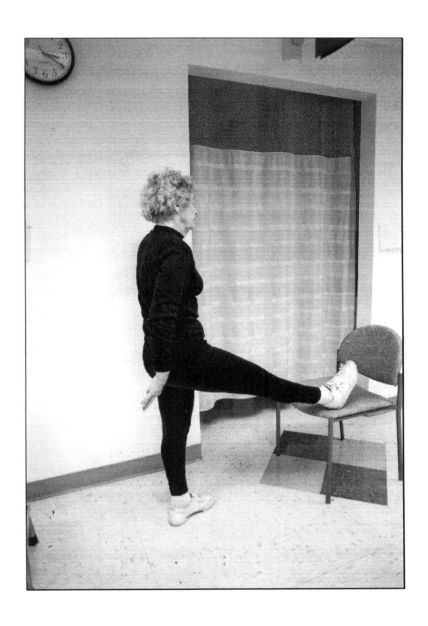

Stand next to a counter or wall for support and balance. Place your foot on a chair or stool. Keep your hips square. Do not let your spine rotate. Keep your knee straight and your foot pointed toward the ceiling. You should feel a stretch behind your knee. Hold 30 seconds and repeat on each leg.

49

STANDING HIP EXTENSION

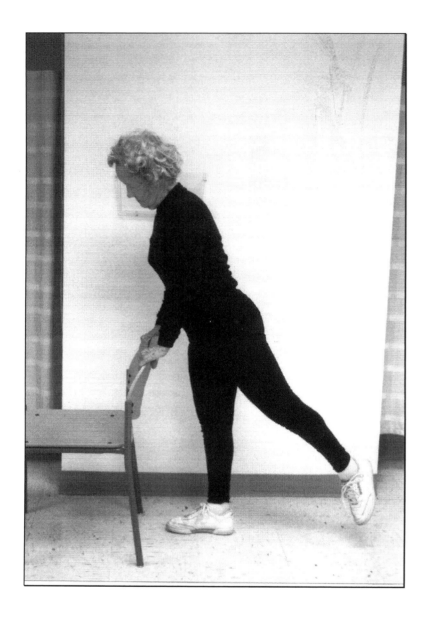

Stand up tall and hold the back of a chair or counter top. Inhale and as you exhale, extend one leg back with a straight knee and lift foot up 2-3" off the floor. Keep the torso steady and avoid leaning forward. Hold 5 seconds an repeat 10 times.

50

ARM RAISES AGAINST A WALL

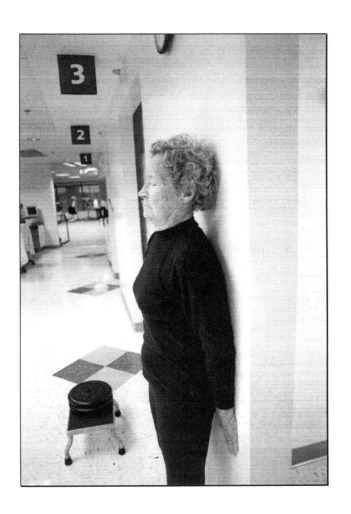 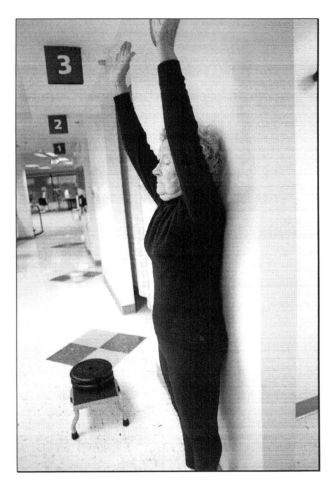

Stand with your hips and head against a wall. Your feet should be about 1 foot in front of the wall. Try to look down while keeping your head against the wall. Inhale and as you exhale, raise both arms as high as you can keeping your shoulders down while maintaining your head position. Hold 5 seconds and repeat 10 times.

51

DOORWAY STRETCH

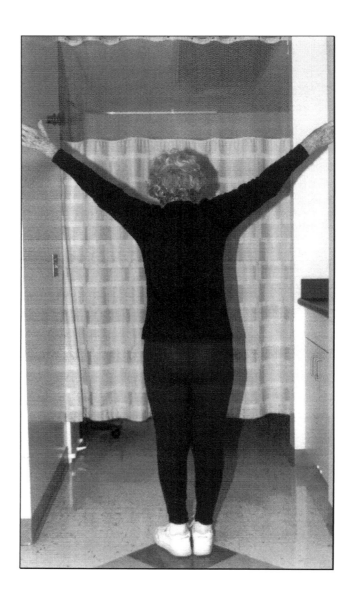

Stand in a doorway. Place both hands as high as possible on each side of the doorframe. Lean your chest forward. Feel the stretch under the arms and across the chest. Hold 30 seconds. Practice deep breathing.

52

CORNER CHEST STRETCH

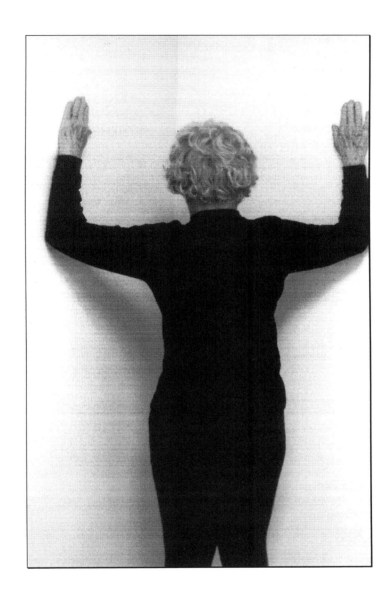

Stand in a corner. Place both hands up on both walls. Elbows are parallel to the ground. Keep elbows against the wall and lean your chest towards the wall. Feel the stretch across your chest. Hold 30 seconds. Practice deep breathing.

"T" EXERCISE STANDING

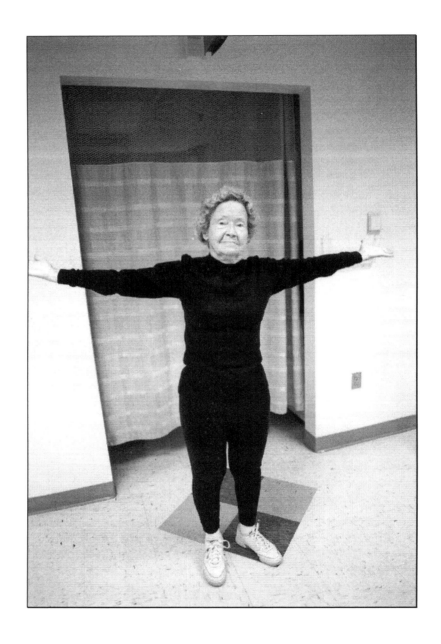

Stand up tall. Hold your hands out in front of you with palms upward. Inhale
and exhale as you open your arms as far as you can with elbows straight.
Draw shoulder blades together. Hold 5 seconds and repeat 10 times.

WALL SLIDES

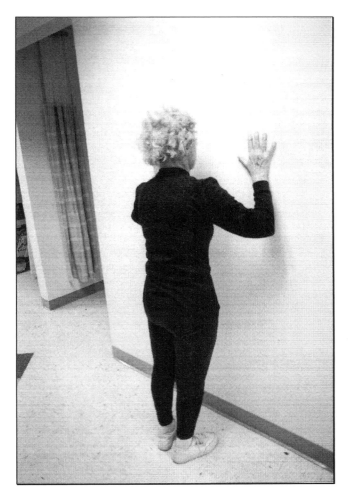 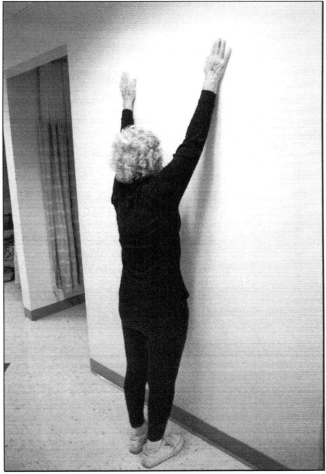

Place both hands up on a wall. Slide your hands up the wall as high as possible. Lean towards the wall. Feel a stretch under the arms. Hold 5 seconds and repeat 10 times. Practice deep breathing.

STANDING PELVIC TILT

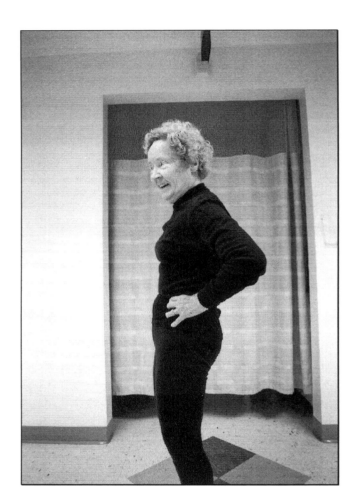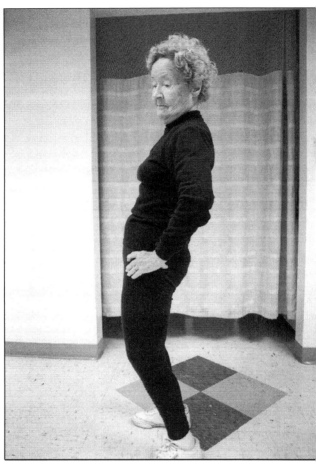

Stand up tall with your hands on your hips. Tighten your buttocks and draw
your abdominals in. Attempt to bring your hip bones toward your ribcage.
Hold 5 seconds. Repeat 10 times.

56

PELVIC CLOCK

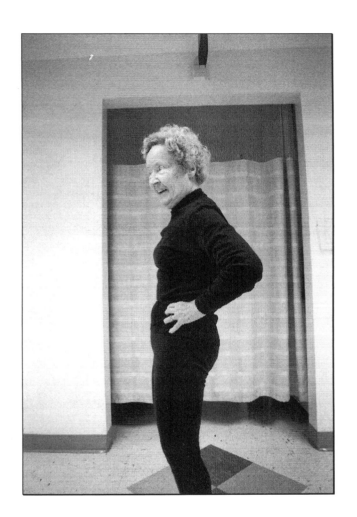

12:00

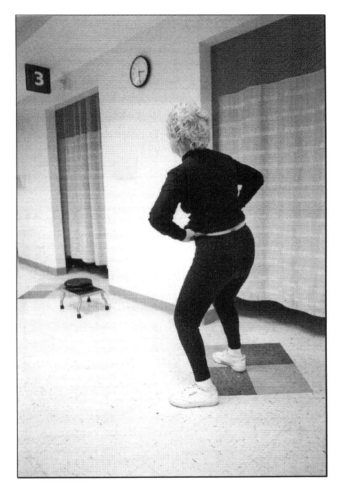

3:00

Stand up tall with your hands on your hips. Imagine that you are the center of a clock. Move your hips straight forward to the 12:00 position, to the right for the 3:00 position, straight back for the 6:00 position, and to the left for the 9:00 position. Repeat 10 times and reverse.

57

PELVIC CLOCK, CONTINUED

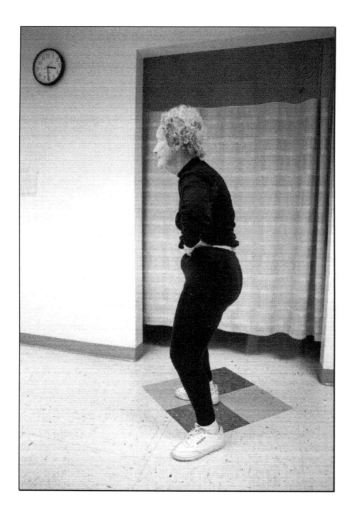

6:00

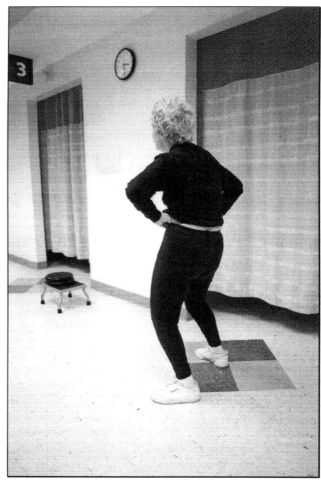

9:00

58

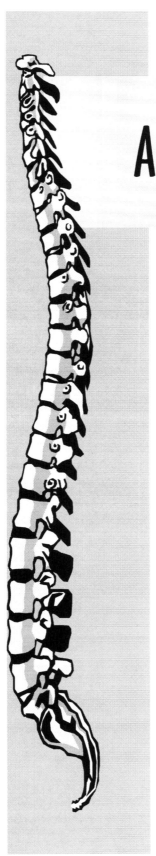

Advanced Level Exercises

SINGLE ARM RAISES WITH WEIGHT

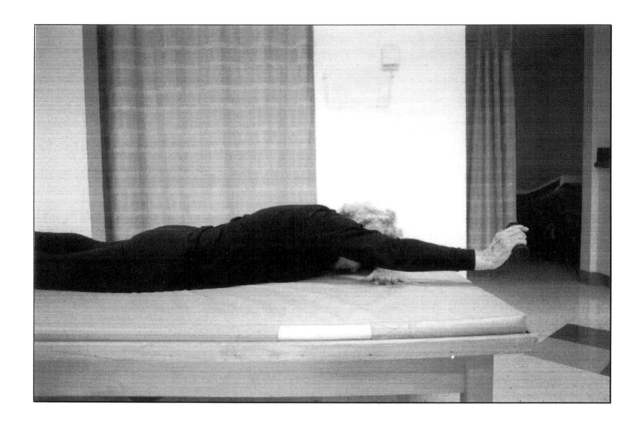

Place your left hand under your forehead with the palm down. Reach your right arm straight out. Grasp the weight. Inhale and as you exhale, raise it up 2-3" off the floor. Hold 5 seconds and repeat 10 times.

"W" EXERCISE WITH WEIGHTS

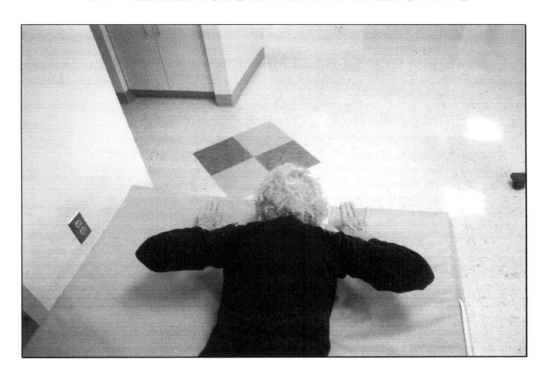

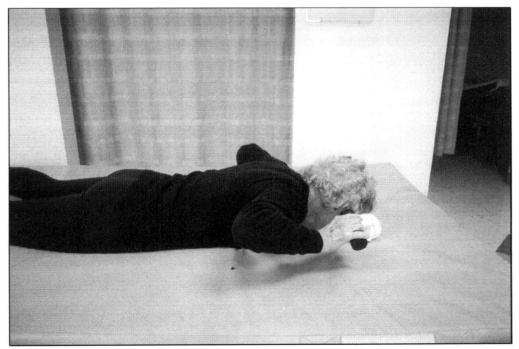

Lie on your stomach with a towel roll under your forehead. Place your hands by your ears. Inhale, and as you exhale, lift the weights and your elbows off the mat. Draw your shoulder blades together and down. Hold 5 seconds and repeat 10 times.

61

PRONE BACK EXTENSION

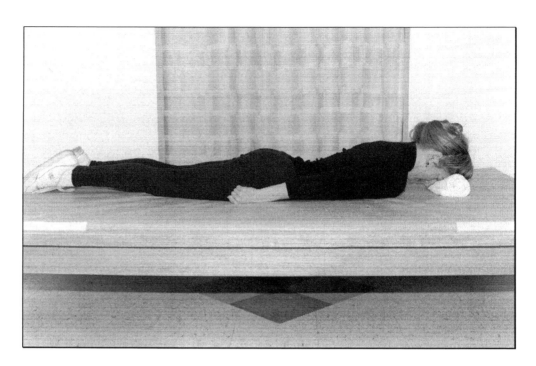

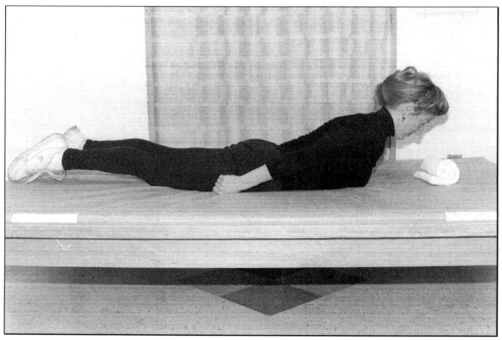

Lie on your stomach with a towel roll under your forehead. Place your arms at your sides. Inhale, keeping your chin down and exhale as you lift your chest off the floor. Draw your shoulder blades down and back. Reach for down the sides of your legs. Hold 5 seconds and repeat 10 times.

62

PRONE "W" EXTENSION

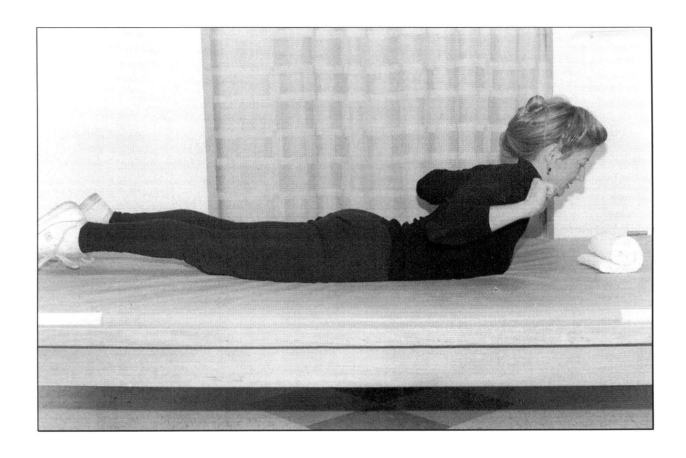

Lie on your stomach with a towel roll under your forehead. Place your arms
in the "W" position with hands by your ears. Inhale, keeping your chin down
and exhale as you lift your chest off the floor. Draw your shoulder blades
down and back. Hold 5 seconds and repeat 10 times.

63

PRONE "T" EXTENSION

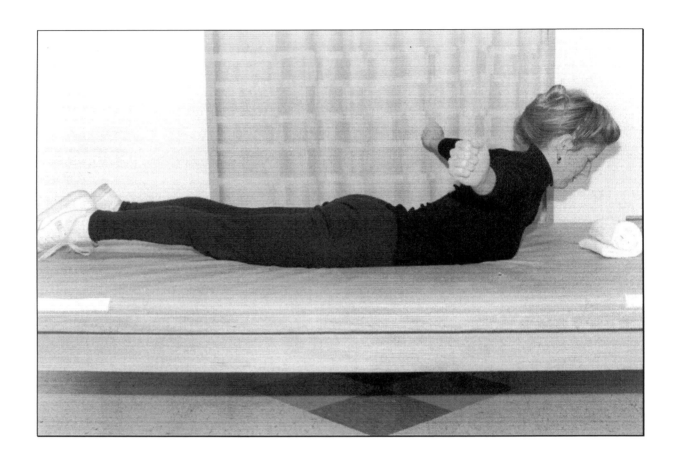

Lie on your stomach with a towel roll under your forehead. Place your arms in the "T" position with arms straight out (like flying). Inhale, keeping your chin down and exhale as you lift your chest off the floor. Draw your shoulder blades down and back. Hold 5 seconds and repeat 10 times.

64

PRONE EXTENSION WITH ARMS OVERHEAD

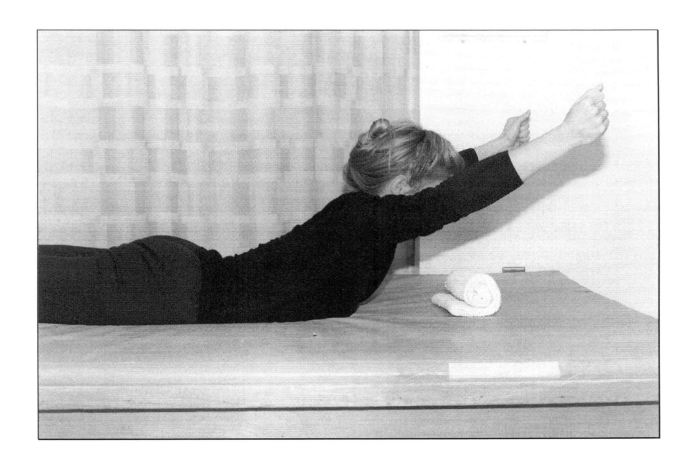

Lie on your stomach with a towel roll under your forehead. Reach your arms overhead (Superman pose). Inhale, keeping your chin down and exhale as you lift your chest off the floor. Draw your shoulder blades down and back. Hold 5 seconds and repeat 10 times.

PRONE BILATERAL HIP EXTENSION

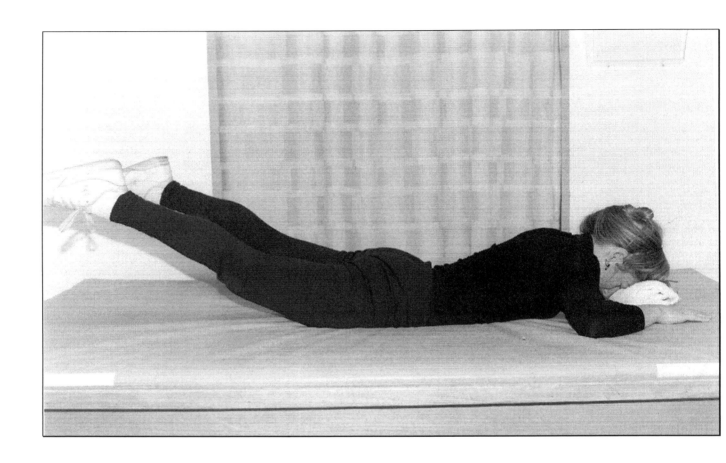

Lie on your stomach with both hands palm down or with a towel under your forehead. Raise both legs off the bed without arching your back. Try to raise your legs with the knees straight. Think of drawing the tailbone down. Hold 5 seconds and repeat 10 times.

PRONE BILATERAL ARM/LEG RAISES

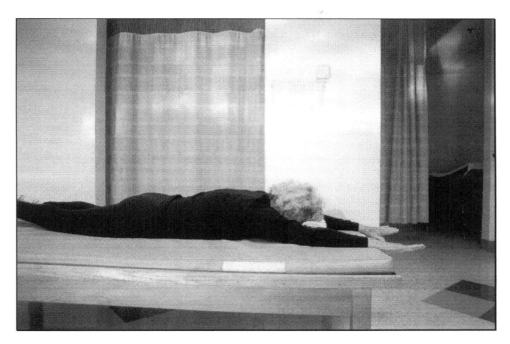

Start with a towel roll under your forehead.

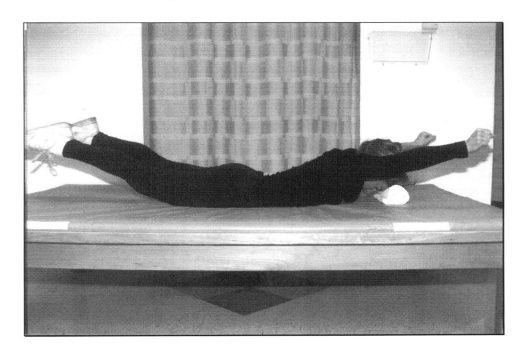

Inhale, and reach both arms and legs straight out and as you exhale, lift them 2-3" with elbows and knees straight. Hold 5 seconds and repeat 10 times.

ALL 4'S BACK ARCHES

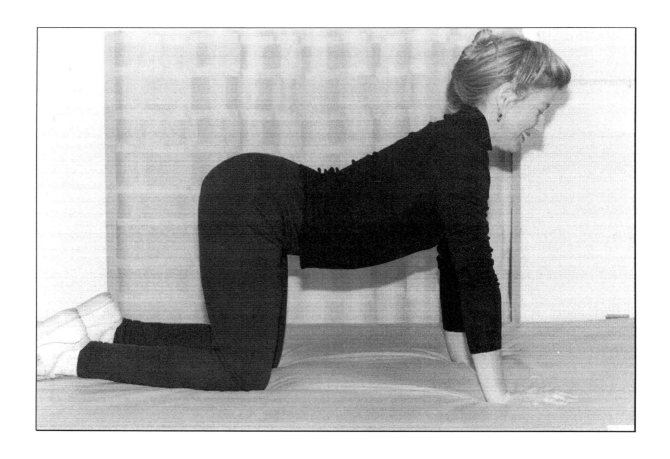

Get in all 4's position. Keep your elbows straight. Sink your stomach toward the floor and try to stick your buttocks out and up. Inhale to lift your breastbone up. Then do a pelvic tilt and round your low back only as you exhale. Aim your lower spine toward the ceiling. Keep your shoulder blades pulled down and back. *Avoid the "angry cat" position!* Repeat 10 times slowly.

ALL 4'S ARM RAISES

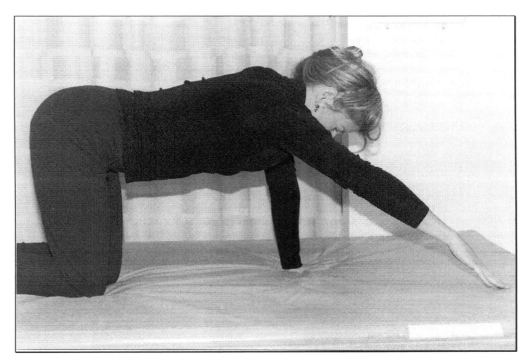

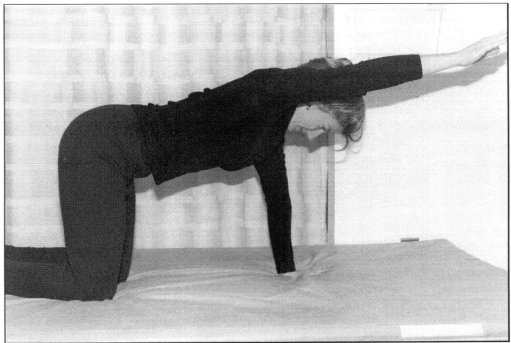

Get in all 4's position. Place your knees under your hips and your hands under your shoulders. Keep your elbows straight. Inhale, and as you exhale, raise one arm up. Keep your spine very still. Hold 5 seconds and repeat 10 times.

ALL 4'S LEG RAISES

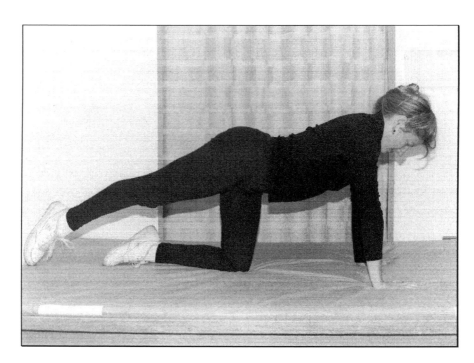

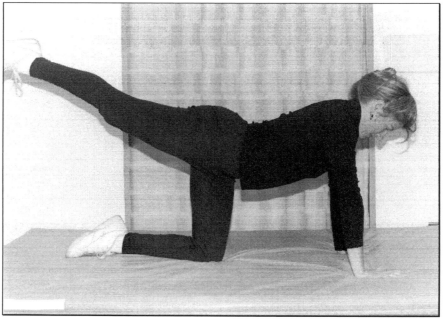

Get in all 4's position. Place your knees under your hips and your hands under your shoulders. Keep your elbows straight and your spine steady. Inhale and extend one leg behind you until the knee is straight. Exhale to raise the leg up. Keep the knee straight. Hold 5 seconds and repeat 10 times.

70

ALL 4'S OPPOSITE ARM/LEG RAISES

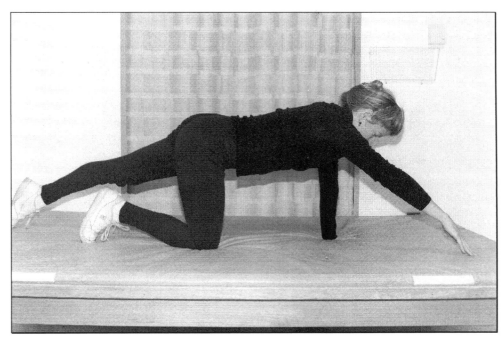

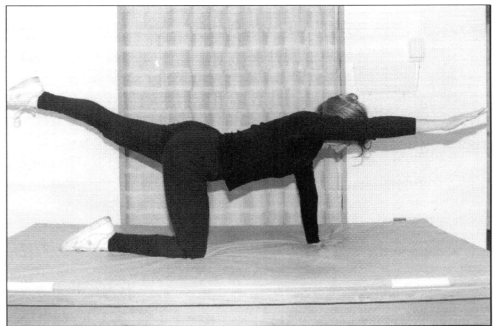

Get in all 4's position. Place your knees under your hips and your hands
under your shoulders. Keep your elbows straight and your spine steady.
Inhale and extend one leg behind you and the opposite arm in front of you.
Exhale, drawing your shoulder blade down and raise the arm and leg up.
Keep the knee and elbow straight. Balance, hold 5 seconds and repeat 10 x.

71

ADVANCED ABDOMINAL EXERCISE

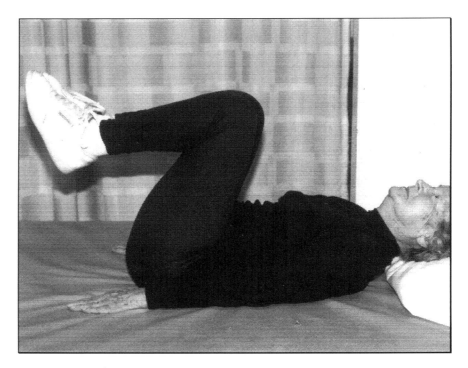

Lie on your back. Bring both knees toward the chest as you inhale.

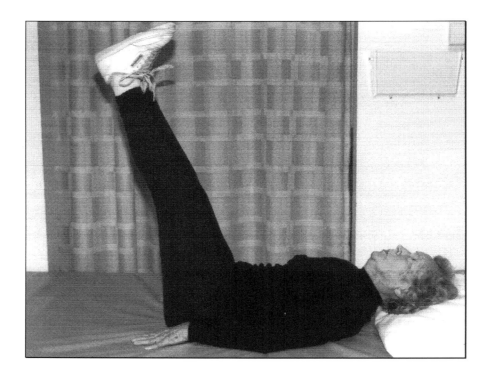

Exhale as you extend both knees until the legs are straight.

72

ADVANCED ABDOMINAL EXERCISE CONTINUED

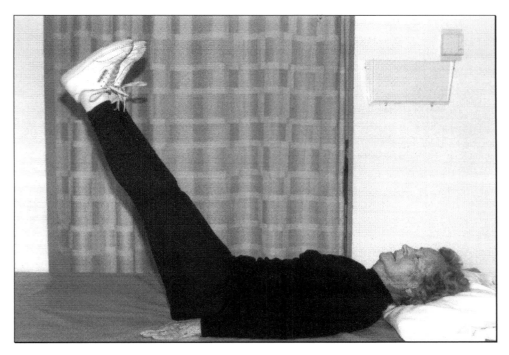

With both hands under the buttocks lower both legs toward the floor.
<u>Keep your low back in contact with the floor</u> and keep the abdominals tight.

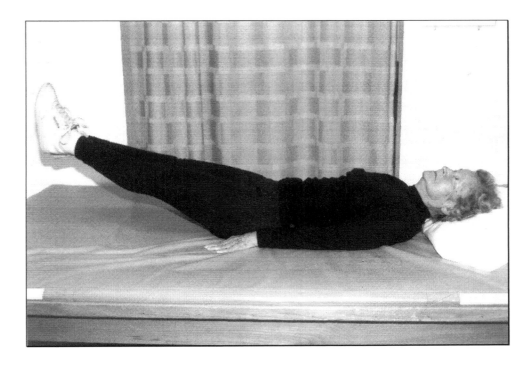

Cntinue to exhale and lower slowly down.(If you lose the pelvic tilt and your
back rises up, or you have any back/neck pain, <u>stop</u> and put your feet down!)

"T" EXERCISE WITH THERABAND

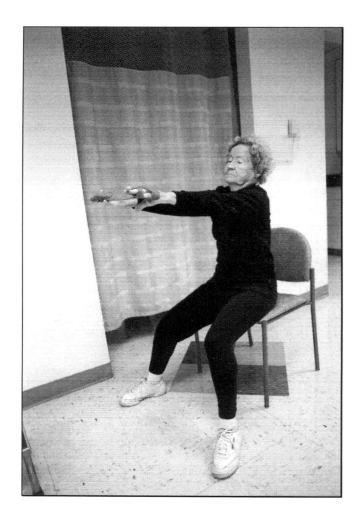 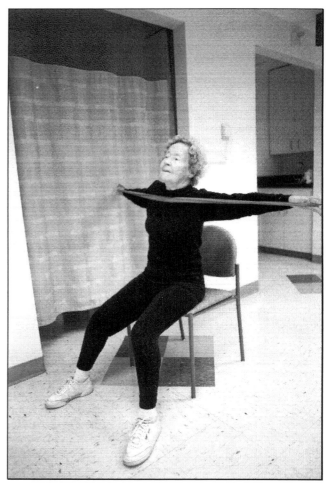

Sit in a chair. Hold a theraband out in front of you with palms upward.
Inhale and as you exhale, pull apart as far as you can with elbows straight.
Draw the shoulder blades together. Hold 5 seconds and repeat 10 times.

74

THERABAND "T" EXERCISE STANDING

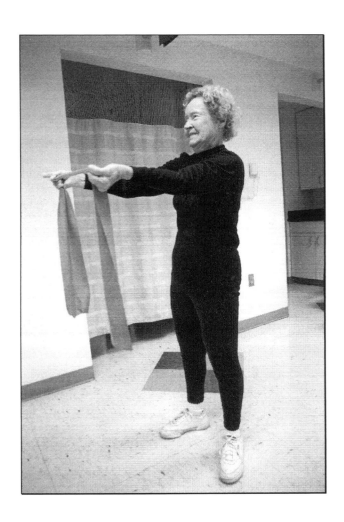 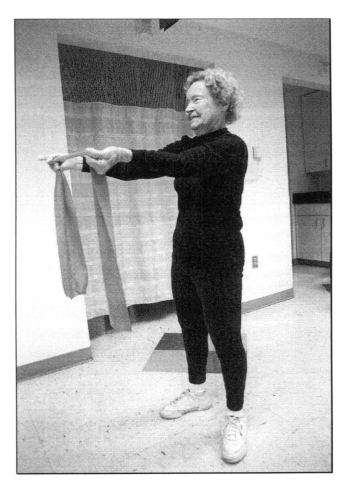

Stand and hold a theraband out in front of you with palms upward. Inhale, and as you exhale, pull apart as far as you can with elbows straight. Draw the shoulder blades together. Hold 5 seconds and repeat 10 times.

75

DIAGONAL THERABAND EXERCISE

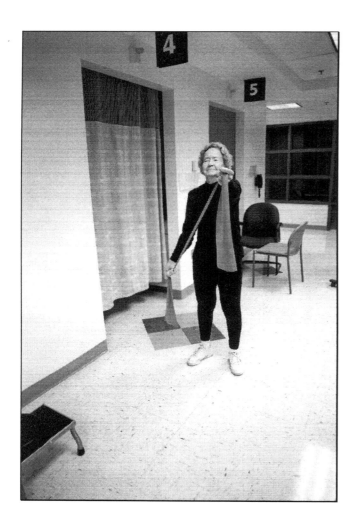 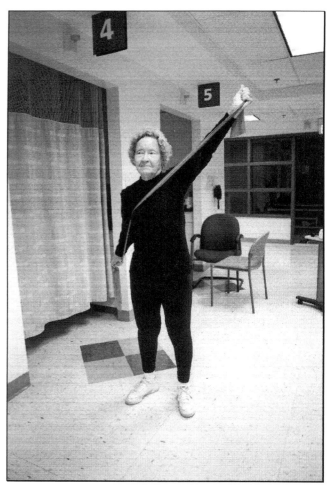

Hold a theraband out in front of you with palms upward. Inhale and as you exhale, pull the left arm up and the right arm down. Hold 5 seconds and repeat 10 times. Then repeat with the right arm up and the left arm down.

76

THERABAND "W" EXERCISE STANDING

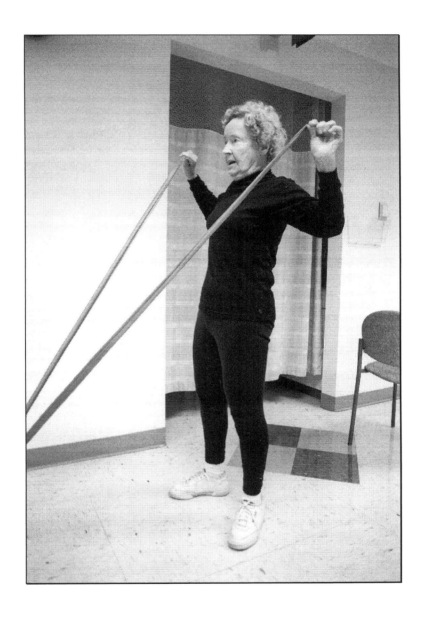

Tie a theraband to a bedpost. Stand and grasp theraband in both hands. Inhale and as you exhale, pull hands up towards your ears. Draw shoulder blades down and back and keep elbows down. Hold 5 seconds and repeat 10 times.

77

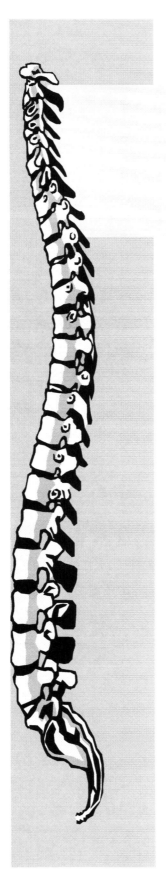

Preventing Fractures

PREVENTING FALLS

LIGHTING:
1. When leaving or entering any room, always turn on the closest light.
2. Use nightlights in dim areas.
3. Use proper illumination of all outdoor exits and walkways.
4. Wear sunglasses to reduce glare on sunny, snowy or icy days.

FLOORS:
1. Remove all throw rugs from your home.
2. Securely fasten edges of all carpeting.
3. Install carpeting on all stairways, being sure it is tacked down well on all edges. This will provide additional cushioning to decrease the risk of fractures or injuries if falls occur.
4. Clear walkways of any stray objects that could cause tripping. Tape electrical cords to the wall or baseboards. Bind any extra cord with a rubber band.
5. Always clean up spills immediately.

BATHROOMS:
1. Install grab bars in the shower or tub area and next to the toilet.
2. Use non-skid strips or mats in the tub and shower floors.
3. Consider using a tub bench or shower chair to make bathing easier and safer.
4. When entering and exiting the tub, sit on the side of the tub and lift your legs over the edge of the tub. Use the grab bars to lower yourself into the tub.
5. Do not use bath oils in your bathtub or shower. The oils cause the surface of the tub to be very slippery.

FOOTWEAR:
1. Do not wear high-heeled shoes. Heels should be no higher than 1 inch.
2. Use shoes with rubber or soft, skid resistant soles that have a wide heel.
3. House slippers should have rubber or non-skid soles. Do not use slippers with a fabric bottom.
4. Do not wear socks on wood or waxed floors.

GENERAL FALL PREVENTION:
1. Do not climb on chairs to reach high objects. Use a sturdy stepladder.
2. Place telephones close to your bed, living area and kitchen. The bathroom is where falls frequently occur and is an excellent place to install a telephone. Don't hurry to answer the telephone, or get caller ID so you can call right back if you are unable to reach the phone in time.
3. Do not get out of bed or get up from a lying position too quickly. Blood pressure is lower in this position and the rapid change can cause dizziness or loss of balance.
4. Speak to your doctor about the drugs you may be taking. Side effects of certain drugs can affect your balance and coordination.
5. Use an assistive device such as a walker or cane if you are uncomfortable in unfamiliar environments. Consult a physical therapist or your physician if you have questions or concerns about assistive devices for walking.

COUGHING AND SNEEZING

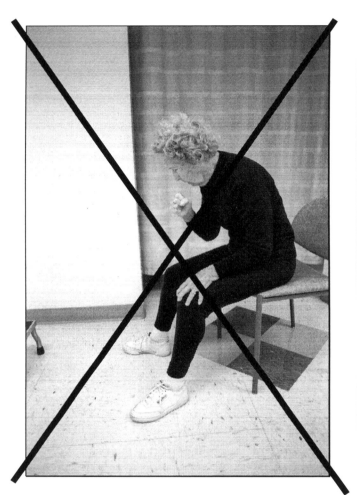 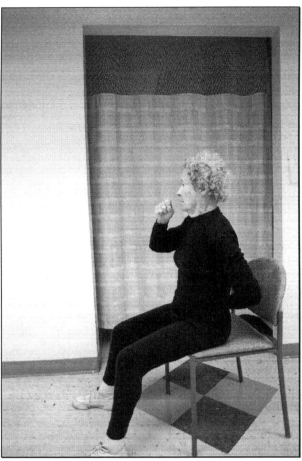

When coughing or sneezing: Do not bend forward! This greatly increases your risk for spinal fractures. Sit up tall with one hand behind your back to cough or sneeze. Keep your back as straight as possible and do not look down. You can lean against a wall or lean back against your chair.

82

REACHING INTO THE OVEN

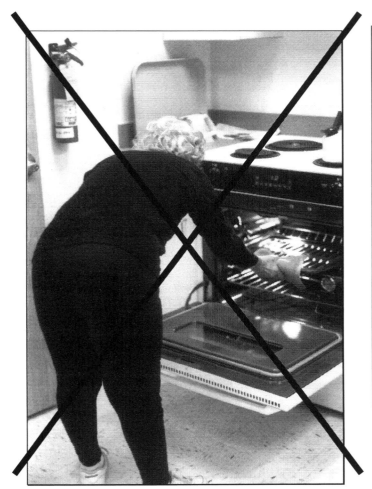 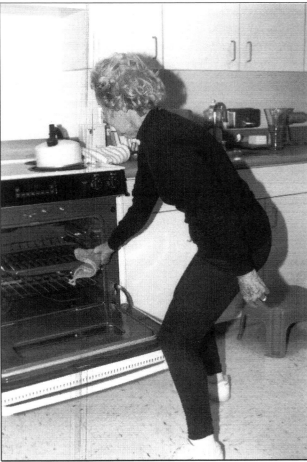

Stand to the side of the oven and bend at the hip without twisting to reach into the oven. Do not stand in front of the oven and try to reach into it.

83

PUTTING ON SHOES

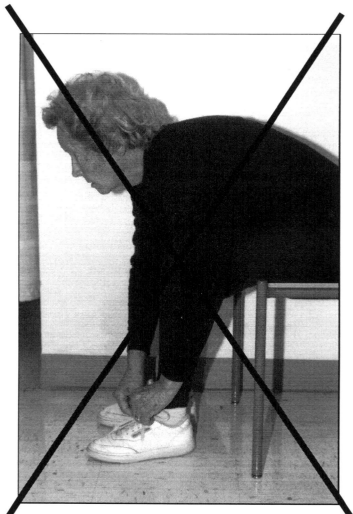 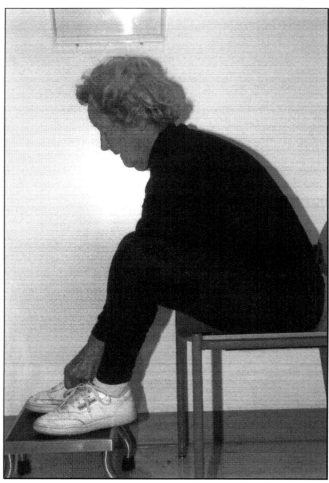

Do not bend forward to put your shoes on. Wear loafers with good support, use a long-handled shoe horn or prop your feet on a stool to put your shoes on. Remember to keep your back straight and bend at the <u>hip</u> to put your shoes on.

84

BRUSHING TEETH & WASHING FACE

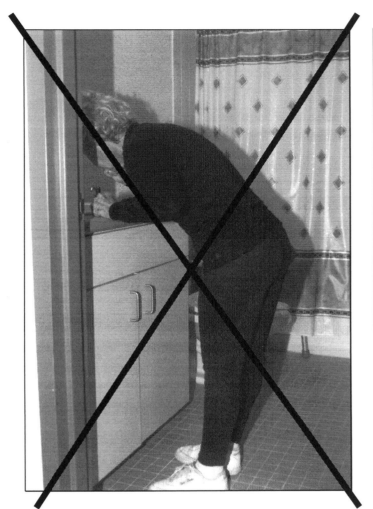 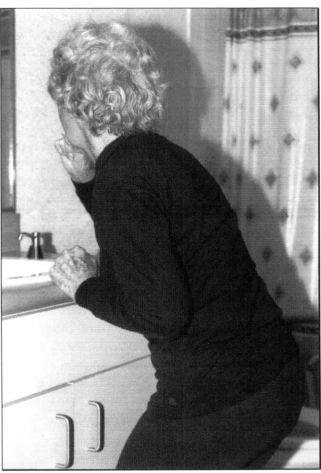

Bend the knees and bend at the hip to brush your teeth or wash your face.
Stand up straight while brushing your teeth. Use a cup to rinse your mouth.
Or to challenge and improve your balance, stand on 1 leg while brushing!

85

USING THE TOILET

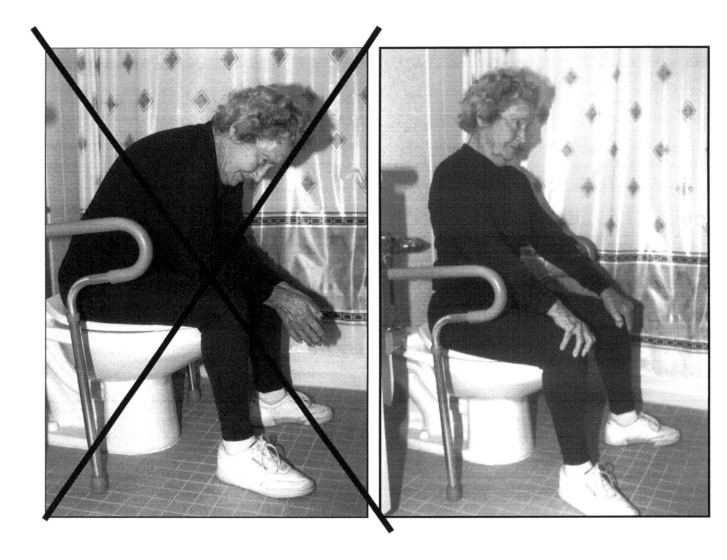

Do not bend forward or slump when using the toilet. Bending forward and rounding the back greatly increases your risk of spine fractures.

Sit up tall with the back as straight as possible when having bowel movements. You can also place both hands on your knees with straight elbows to provide extra support.

86

PARTIAL SQUAT

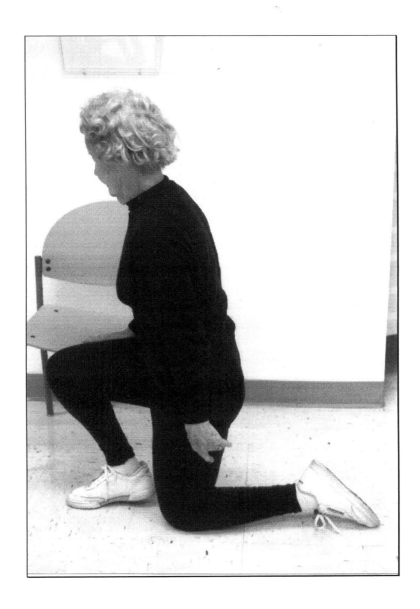

Use a chair or some type of support and place one foot in front of the other. Slowly lower yourself down to one knee. Return to standing without bending forward. Repeat 10 times. This activity will enable you to get down far enough to reach into low cabinets or to pick things up off the floor if you are unable to do a full squat or have a knee problem.

FULL SQUAT

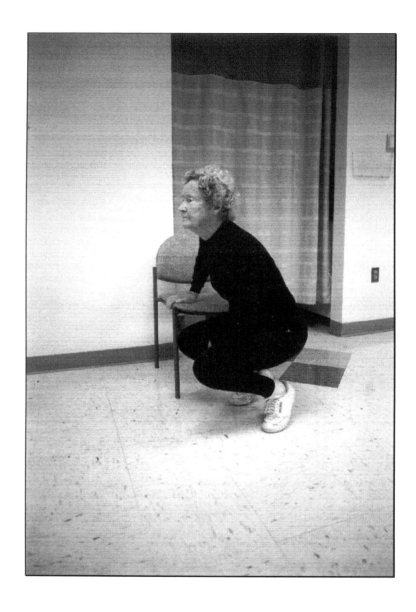

Use a chair or some type of support and slowly lower yourself down until your buttocks come close to your heels. Slowly return to standing. Repeat 10 times. This activity will enable you to get down far enough to reach into low cabinets or to pick things up off the floor. Also keeps the hip, knee and ankle joints fully mobile!

REFERENCES

Aloia JF, et. al., "Premenopausal bone mass is related to physical activity." *Archives of Internal Medicine* 1988;148:121-123.

Andrade SE, Majumdar SR, Chan KA, Buist DS, Go AS, Goodman M, Smith DH, Platt R, Gurwitz JH. Low frequency of treatment of osteoporosis among postmenopausal women following a fracture. *Arch Intern Med.* 2003 Sep 22;163(17):2052-7.

Ayalon J, et. al. "Dynamic bone-loading exercises for postmenopausal osteoporotic women: effect on the density of the distal radius." *Arch Phys Med Rehab* 1987;68:280-283.

Bailey DA, et. al., "Physical activity, nutrition, bone density and osteoporosis." *Australian J of Science and Medicine in Sport* 1986;18:3-8.

Bassey EJ, et. al., "Increase in femoral bone density in young women following high-impact exercise." *Osteoporosis International* 1994;4:72-75.

Bassey, EJ, "Exercise for prevention of osteoporotic fracture." *Age and Aging* 2001; 30 (Suppl. 4), 29-31.

Bauer JJ, Snow CM. "What is the prescription for healthy bones?" *J Musculoskelet Neuronal Interact.* 2003 Dec;3(4):352-5; discussion 356.

Beck BR, Snow CM. "Bone health across the lifespan--exercising our options." *Exerc Sport Sci Rev.* 2003 Jul;31(3):117-22. (Review)

Beverly, et. al., "Local bone mineral response to brief exercise that stresses the skeleton." *British Med J* 1989;299:233-235.

Betz SR. "Modifying Pilates for Osteoporosis." *Idea Fitness Journal* 2007 Apr;47-55.

Block JE, et. al., "Does exercise prevent osteoporosis? *JAMA* 1987;257:3115-17.

Bonner EJ, et. al., "Health Professional's guide to rehabilitation of the patient with osteoporosis." *Osteoporosis International*, 14 (Suppl. 2), S1-22.

Bonnick SL. *The Osteoporosis Handbook.* Taylor Publishing: Dallas, TX, 1997.

Bouxsein ML, et. al., "Overview of exercise and bone mass." *Osteoporosis* 1994;20:787-802.

Briggs AM, Greig AM, Wark JD, Fazzalari NL, Bennell KL. "A review of anatomical and mechanical factors affecting vertebral body integrity." *Int J Med Sci.* 2004;1(3):170-180.

Briggs AM, Wark JD, Kantor S, Fazzalari NL, Greig AM, Bennell KL. "Bone mineral density distribution in thoracic and lumbar vertebrae: an ex vivo study using dual energy X-ray absorptiometry." *Bone*. 2006 Feb;38(2):286-8.

Briggs AM, et al. The effect of osteoporotic vertebral fracture on predicted spinal loads in vivo. *Eur Spine J*. 2006; 15:1785–1795

Briggs AM, et. al. The vertebral fracture cascade in osteoporosis: a review of aetiopathogenesis. *Osteoporosis International*. 2007 May;18(5):575-84.

Briggs AM, Greig AM, Wark JD. "The vertebral fracture cascade in osteoporosis: a review of aetiopathogenesis." *Osteoporos Int*. 2007 May;18(5):575-84. (Review)

Briggs AM, et al. "Thoracic kyphosis affects spinal loads and trunk muscle force." *Phys Ther*. 2007 May;87(5):595-607.

Briggs AM, et. al. Paraspinal muscle control in people with osteoporotic vertebral fracture. *European Spine Journal* 2007 Aug;16(8):1137-44..

Campbell TC. *The China Study*. Benbella Books: Dallas, 2005.

Cardinale M, Rittweger J. Vibration exercise makes your muscles and bones stronger: fact or fiction? *J Br Menopause Soc*. 2006 Mar;12(1):12-8.

Carter, "Mechanical loading history and skeletal biology." *J of Biomechanics* 1987;20:1095-1109.

Cavanaugh JT, Shinberg M, Ray L, Shipp KM, Kuchibhatla M, Schenkman M. "Kinematic characterization of standing reach: comparison of younger vs. older subjects." *Clin Biomech* (Bristol, Avon) 1999 May;14(4):271-9.

Chalmers J, Ho KC, "Geographical variations in senile osteoporosis. The association with physical activity." *J Bone Joint Surg* 1970, 52B:667-75.

Chan K, Qin L, Lau M, Woo J, Au S, Choy W, Lee K, Lee S. A randomized, prospective study of the effects of Tai Chi Chun exercise on bone mineral density in postmenopausal women. *Arch Phys Med Rehabil*. 2004 May;85(5):717-22.

Chow R, Harrison JE, and Notarius C, "Effect of two randomized exercise programmes on bone mass of healthy post-menopausal women." Br Med J 1987; 295:1141-44.

Coletti LA, et. al., "The Effects of Muscle Building Exercise on Bone Mineral Density of the Radius, Spine and Hip in Young Men." *Calcification Tissue International* 1989:45;12-14.

Cooper C, et al. "Review: developmental origins of osteoporotic fracture." *Osteoporos Int*. 2006;17(3):337-47. (Review)

Cowin SC, "Mechanical modeling of the stress adaptation process in bone." *Calcified Tissue International* 1984;36:S98-S103.

Cummings SR, Melton LJ 3rd. Epidemiology and outcomes of osteoporotic fractures. Lancet 2002 May 18;359(9319):1761-7.

Dalsky GA, "The role of exercise in the prevention of osteoporosis." *Comprehensive Therapy* 1989;15:30-37.

Dalsky GP, et. al., "Weight-bearing exercise training and lumbar bone mineral ontent in postmenopausal women." *Ann Int Med* 1988;1008:824-828.

Dalsky GP, "Effect of exercise on bone: permissive influence of estrogen and calcium." *Medicine and Science in Sports and Exercise* 1990;22:281-285.

Davis CM. *Complementary Therapies in Rehabilitation, 2nd. Ed.* Slack Publishing, 2004, Chapter 13: Pilates Rehabilitation by Brent Anderson, PhD, PT, OCS.

Dawson-Hughes B, et. al. "Bone density of the radius, spine and hip in relation to percent of ideal body weight in postmenopausal women." *Calcification Tissue International* 1987;40:310-314.

DeBenedette V, "Study: Swimming may increase bone density." *The Physician and Sports Med* 1987; 15(12):49.

Dontas IA, Yiannakopoulos CK. "Risk factors and prevention of osteoporosis-related fractures." *J Musculoskelet Neuronal Interact.* 2007 Jul-Sep;7(3):268-72. (Review)

Feldstein AC, Nichols GA, Elmer PJ, Smith DH, Aickin M, Herson M. Older women with fractures: Patients falling through the cracks of guideline-recommended osteoporosis screening and treatment. J Bone Joint Surg AM 2003 De;85-A(12):2294-302.

Ferretti JL, Cointry GR, Capozza RF, Frost HM. "Bone mass, bone strength, muscle-bone interactions, osteopenias and osteoporoses." *Mech Ageing Dev.* 2003 Mar;124(3):269-79. (Review)

Fiatarone MA, et. al., "High-intensity strength training in nonagenarians." *JAMA* 1990;263:3029-3024.

Foundation for Osteoporosis Research and Education (FORE). *Guidelines for the Physician (4th Ed.), FORE.*

Francis RM, et al. "Back pain in osteoporotic vertebral fractures." *Osteoporosis Int.* 2007 Dec 11.

Frost HM, "Vital biomechanics:proposed general concepts for skeletal adaptation to mechanical usage." *Calcified Tissue International* 1988;42:145-156.

91

Frost HM. "Coming changes in accepted wisdom about 'osteoporosis'."
J Musculoskelet Neuronal Interact. 2004 Mar;4(1):78-85. (Review)

Fuchs RK, Snow CM. "Gains in hip bone mass from high-impact training are maintained: a randomized controlled trial in children." *J Pediatr.* 2002 Sep;141(3):357-62.

Gaby AR, *Preventing and Reversing Osteoporosis.* Prima Publishing: Rocklin, CA, 1994.

Gass M, Dawson-Hughes B. "Preventing osteoporosis-related fractures: an overview."
Am J Med. 2006 Apr;119(4 Suppl 1):S3-S11. (Review)

Gold DT, Shipp KM, Pieper CF, Duncan PW, Martinez S, Lyles KW. "Group treatment improves trunk strength and psychological status in older women with vertebral fractures: results of a randomized, clinical trial.' *J Am Geriatr Soc.* 2004 Sep;52(9):1471-8.

Gold DT, Shipp KM, Lyles KW. "Managing patients with complications of osteoporosis."
Endocrinol Metab Clin North Am. 1998 Jun;27(2):485-96. (Review)

Goldstein E, Simkin A, "The influence of weight-bearing water exercise on bone density of post-menopausal women. Movement-" *J of Physical Education and Sport Sciences*(Heb.) 1994;2:7-30.

Gordon-Larson P, Mc Murray RG, Popkin BM. Adolescent physical activity and inactivity vary by ethnicity: The National Longitudinal Study of Adolescent Health. *J Pediatr* 1999 Sep;135(3):301-6.

Granhead H, Jonson R, Hansson T, "The loads on the lumbar spine during extreme weight-lifting." *Spine* 1987;12:146-149.

Greig AM, Bennell KL, Briggs AM, Hodges PW. "Postural taping decreases thoracic kyphosis but does not influence trunk muscle electromyographic activity or balance in women with osteoporosis." *Man Ther.* 2007 Apr 11.

Greig AM, Bennell KL, Briggs AM, Wark JD, Hodges PW. "Balance impairment is related to vertebral fracture rather than thoracic kyphosis in individuals with osteoporosis."
Osteoporos Int. 2007 Apr;18(4):543-51.

Grote HJ, et. al., "Intervertebral variation in trabecular microarchitecture throughout the normal spine in relation to age." *Bone*, 1995; 116(3), 301-8.

Hingorjo MR, et al. "Role of exercise in osteoporosis prevention--current concepts."
J Pak Med Assoc. 2008 Feb;58(2):78-81.

Holick MF, et al. "Prevalence of Vitamin D inadequacy among postmenopausal North American women receiving osteoporosis therapy." *J Clin Endocrinol Metab.* 2005 Jun;90(6):3215-24.

Hongo M, Itoi E, Sinaki M, et al. "Effect of low-intensity back exercise on quality of life and back extensor strength in patients with osteoporosis: a randomized controlled trial." *Osteoporos Int*. 2007 Oct;18(10):1389-95.

Hourigan SR, Nitz JC, Brauer SG, O'Neill S, Wong J, Richardson CA. "Positive effects of exercise on falls and fracture risk in osteopenic women." *Osteoporos Int*. 2008 Jan 11.

Hu JF, et. al., "Bone density and lifestyle characteristics in premenopausal and postmenopausal Chinese women (part of the China-Cornell Project). *Osteoporosis International,* 1994; 4(6), 288-97.

Huntoon E, Sinaki M. "Thoracic osteoporotic fracture without upper back pain." *Am J Phys Med Rehabil*. 2004 Sep;83(9):729.

Huntoon EA, Sinaki M. "The role of exercise in the prevention and treatment of compression fractures." *Mayo Clin Proc*. 2006 Oct;81(10):1400; author reply 1400-1.

Huntoon EA, Schmidt CK, Sinaki M. "Significantly fewer refractures after vertebroplasty in patients who engage in back-extensor-strengthening exercises." *Mayo Clin Proc*. 2008 Jan;83(1):54-7.

Kasper MJ, "Can vigorous exercise play a role in osteoporosis prevention?" *Osteoporosis International* 1992;2:55-69.

Kanders B, Dempster D, Lindsay R, "Interaction of calcium, nutrition and physical activity on bone mass in young women." *J Bone Min Res* 1988;3:145-149.

Keller TS, et. al., Prediction of Spinal Deformity. *Spine*, 2003; 28(5), 455-62.

Kiebzak GM, Beinart GA, Perser K, Ambrose CG, Siff SJ, Heggeness MH. Undertreatment of osteoporosis in men with hip fracture. *Arch Intern Med*. 2002; Oct 28;162(19):2217-22.

Kohrt WM, et. al., "Additive effects of weight-bearing exercises and estrogen on bone mineral density in older women. *J Bone Min Res* 1995;10:1303-1311.

Kruk J. "Physical activity in the prevention of the most frequent chronic diseases: an analysis of the recent evidence." *Asian Pac J Cancer Prev*. 2007 Jul-Sep;8(3):325-38.

Lane NE, et al, "Long distance running, bone density and osteoarthritis." *JAMA* 1986; 255:1147-51.

Lanyon LE. "Functional strain as determinant of bone remodeling." *Calcified Tissue International* 1984;36:S56-S61.

Lanyon LE, "Functional strain in bone tissue as objective, and controlling stimulus for adaptive bone remodeling." *Journal of Biomechanics* 1987;20:1083-93.

93

Larson KA, et. al., "Decreasing the incidence of osteoporosis-related injuries through diet and exercise. *Public Health Reports* 1984;99:609-613.
LeBlanc A, et. al., "Spinal bone mineral after 5 weeks of bed rest." *Calcification Tissue International* 1987;41:259-261.

Leichter I, Simkin A, et. al. "Gain in mass density of bone following strenuous physical activity." *J Ortho Res* 1989;1:86-90.

Lin JT, Lane JM. "Rehabilitation of the older adult with an osteoporosis-related fracture." *Clin Geriatr Med.* 2006 May;22(2):435-47. (Review)

Lindsay R, et. al., "Risk of a new vertebral fracture in the year following a fracture." JAMA 2001; 285 (3), 320-3.

Liu-Ambrose TY, et al. "The beneficial effects of group-based exercises on fall risk profile and physical activity persist 1 year post intervention in older women with low bone mass: follow-up after withdrawal of exercise." *J Am Geriatr Soc.* 2005 Oct;53(10):1767-73.

Lui PP, Qin L, Chan KM. "Tai Chi Chuan exercises in enhancing bone mineral density in active seniors." *Clin Sports Med.* 2008 Jan;27(1):75-86, viii. (Review)

Lyles KW, Gold DT, Shipp KM, Pieper CF, Martinez S, Mulhausen PL. "Association of osteoporotic vertebral compression fractures with impaired functional status." *Am J Med.* 1993 Jun;94(6):595-601.

Maciaszek J, et al. "Effect of Tai Chi on body balance: randomized controlled trial in men with osteopenia or osteoporosis." *Am J Chin Med.* 2007;35(1):1-9.

Maddalozzo GF, Widrick JJ, Cardinal BJ, Winters-Stone KM, Hoffman MA, Snow CM. "The effects of hormone replacement therapy and resistance training on spine bone mineral density in early postmenopausal women." *Bone.* 2007 May;40(5):1244-51.

Madureira MM, et al. "Balance training program is highly effective in improving functional status and reducing the risk of falls in elderly women with osteoporosis: a randomized controlled trial." *Osteoporos Int.* 2007 Apr;18(4):419-25.

Martyn-St James M, Carroll S. "High-intensity resistance training and postmenopausal bone loss: a meta-analysis." *Osteoporos Int.* 2006;17(8):1225-40.

Meeks S, *Walk Tall! An Exercise Program for the Prevention and Treatment of Osteoporosis.* Triad Publishing, 1999.

Meeks, S. The role of the Physical Therapist in the Recognition, Assessment and Exercise Intervention in Persons with, or at risk for, Osteoporosis. Topics in Geriatric Rehabilitation, Oct 2004.

Metz JA, Anderson JJ, Gallagher PN Jr, "Intakes of calcium, phosphorus and protein, and physical activity level are related to radial bone mass in young adult women" *Am J Clin Nutr* 1993 Oct;58(4):537-42.

Michel BA, Bloch DA, Fries JF. Weight-bearing exercise, overexercise, and lumbar bone density over age 50 years. Arch Intern Med. 1989 Oct;149(10):2325-9.

Mosekdile L, "Osteoporosis and Exercise (Editorial). *Bone* 1995;17:193-195.

National Osteoporosis Foundation. America's Bone Health: The State of Osteoporosis and Low Bone Mass in Our Nation. Washington, DC: NOF; 2002.

Nattiv A, et al. "American College of Sports Medicine position stand. The female athlete triad." *Med Sci Sports Exerc.* 2007 Oct;39(10):1867-82.

Nelson ME, *Strong Women Stay Young.* Bantam Books: New York, 1997.

Nelson ME, et al, "Diet and bone status in amenorrheic runners." *Am J Clin Nutr* 1986; 43:910-16.

Nelson ME, et. al., "Effects of high intensity strength training on multiple risk factors for osteoporotic fractures-A randomized controlled trial." *JAMA* 1994;272:1909-1914.

North American Menopause Society. "Management of osteoporosis in postmenopausal women: 2006 position statement of The North American Menopause Society." *Menopause* 2006 May-Jun;13(3):340-67; quiz 368-9.

Northrup, Christiane. *Women's Bodies, Women's Wisdom 2nd Ed.* Bantam Books: New York, 1998.

Notelovitz M, et al, *Stand Tall! Every Woman's Guide to Preventing and Treating Osteoporosis.* Triad Publishing, 1998.

Notelovitz M, et. al., "Estrogen therapy and variable resistance weight training increase bone mineral in surgically menopausal women." *J Bone Min Res* 1991;6:583-590.

Orswoll ES, et. al., "The effect of swimming exercises on bone mineral contents." *Clin Res* 1987;35:194A.

Ozdemir F, et al. "Evaluation of the efficacy of therapeutic ultrasound on bone mineral density in postmenopausal period." *Rheumatol Int.* 2008 Feb;28(4):361-5.

Palombaro KM. "Effects of walking-only interventions on bone mineral density at various skeletal sites: a meta-analysis." *J Geriatr Phys Ther.* 2005;28(3):102-7.

Park H, et al. "Relationship of bone health to yearlong physical activity in older Japanese adults: cross-sectional data from the Nakanojo Study." *Osteoporos Int.* 2007 Mar;18(3):285-93.

Pesonen J, et al. "High bone mineral density among perimenopausal women." *Osteoporos Int.* 2005 Dec;16(12):1899-906.

Pfeifer M, Sinaki M, Geusens P, Boonen S, Preisinger E, Minne HW; "ASBMR Working Group on Musculoskeletal Rehabilitation. Musculoskeletal rehabilitation in osteoporosis: a review." *J Bone Miner Res.* 2004 Aug;19(8):1208-14.

Pocock NA, et al, "Physical fitness is a major determinant of femoral neck and lumbar spine bone mineral density." *J Clin Invest* 1986, 78:618-21.

Prince R, Devine A, et al, "The effects of calcium supplementation (milk powder or tablets) and exercise on bone mineral density in postmenopausal women. *J Bone Miner Res* 1995 Jul;10(7):1068-75.

Prince RL, Smith M, et al, "Prevention of postmenopausal osteoporosis. A comparative study of exercise, calcium supplementation, and hormone replacement therapy." *N Engl J Med* 1991 Oct 24;325(17):1189-95.

Pruitt LA, et. al., "Weight-training effects of bone mineral density in early post-menopausal women." *J Bone Min Res* 1992;7:179-185.

Purser JL, Pieper CF, Branch LG, Shipp KM, Gold DT, Lyles KW. "Spinal deformity and mobility self-confidence among women with osteoporosis and vertebral fractures." *Aging (Milano).* 1999 Aug;11(4):235-45.

Revel M, et. al., "One year psoas training can prevent lumbar bone loss in postmenopausal women: A randomized controlled trial." *Calcified Tissue International* 1993;53:307-311.

Reventlow SD. "Perceived risk of osteoporosis: restricted physical activities? Qualitative interview study with women in their sixties." *Scand J Prim Health Care.* 2007 Sep;25(3):160-5.

Riggs BL, Melton LJ 3rd. The worldwide problem of osteoporosis: insights afforded by epidemiology. Bone 1995 Nov; 17 (5 Suppl):505S-11S.

Rittweger J. Can exercise prevent osteoporosis? *J Musculoskelet Neuronal Interact.* 2006 Apr-Jun;6(2):162-6. (Review)

Sakamoto K, Nakamura T, Hagino H, Endo N, Mori S, Muto Y, Harada A, Nakano T, Itoi E, Yoshimura M, Norimatsu H, Yamamoto H, Ochi T; "Committee on Osteoporosis of The Japanese Orthopaedic Association. Effects of unipedal standing balance exercise on the prevention of falls and hip fracture among clinically defined high-risk elderly individuals: a randomized controlled trial." *J Orthop Sci.* 2006 Oct;11(5):467-72.

Salkeld G, Cameron ID, Cumming RG, Easter S, Seymour J, Kurrle SE, Quine S. Quality of life related to fear of falling and hip fracture in older women: A time trade off study. BMJ 2000 Feb 5;320(7231):341-6.

Schapira D, "Physical exercise in the prevention and treatment of osteoporosis-A review. *J of the Royal Society of Medicine* 1988;81:461-63.

Schenkman M, Shipp KM, Chandler J, Studenski SA, Kuchibhatla M. "Relationships between mobility of axial structures and physical performance." *Phys Ther.* 1996 Mar;76(3):276-85.

Schwab P, & Klein RF. "Nonpharmacological approaches to improve bone health and reduce osteoporosis." *Curr Opin Rheumatol.* 2008 Mar;20(2):213-7.

Seeman E. "Loading and bone fragility." *J Bone Miner Metab.* 2005;23 Suppl:23-9. (Review)

Shangold MM, "Exercise in the Menopausal Woman." *Obstetrics and Gynecology* 1990: 75;53s-58s.

Shipp K, Duke University Center for Aging. "Promoting Strong Bones and Vitality Across the Lifespan" Healthcare Professions Seminar, Atlanta, GA, July 1997.

Shipp KM, et al. "Timed loaded standing: a measure of combined trunk and arm endurance suitable for people with vertebral osteoporosis." *Osteoporos Int.* 2000;11(11):914-22.

Shipp KM. "Exercise for people with osteoporosis: translating the science into clinical practice." *Curr Osteoporos Rep.* 2006 Dec;4(4):129-33. (Review)

Sievänen H, & Kannus P. "Physical activity reduces the risk of fragility fracture. *PLoS Med.* 2007 Jun;4(6):e222.

Simkin A, Ayalon J, Leichter I, "Increased trabecular bone density due to bone-loading exercise in postmenopausal osteoporotic women." *Calcification Tissue International* 1987;40:59-63.

Simkin A, et. al., "Arrest of bone loss in middle and late life women by bone-loading physical activity-A community oriented study." Submitted for publication 1995.

Sinaki M, Mikkelsen, BA "Postmenopausal spinal osteoporosis: Flexion versus extension exercises." *Arch Phys Med Rehab* 1984; 65;593-596.

Sinaki M, et. al., Relationship between bone mineral density of spine and strength of back extensors in healthy postmenopausal women. Mayo Clinic Proceedings 1986; 61(2), 116-22.

Sinaki M, "Exercise and Physical Therapy." In *Osteoporosis: Etiology, diagnosis and management*, edited by BL Riggs and LJ Melton, III, Chapter 19, 1988;New York: Raven Press.

Sinaki M, "The role of exercise in preventing osteoporosis." *J Musculo Med* 1992, 67-83.

Sinaki M, Wollan PC, Scott RW, Gelczer RK. Can strong back extensors prevent vertebral fractures in women with osteoporosis? Mayo Clin Proc. 1996 Oct;71(10):951-6.

Sinaki M, et. al., Stronger back musles reduce the incidence of vertebral fracturs: A prospective 10 year follow-up of postmenopausal women. Bone 2002; 30(6), 836-41.

Sinaki M. "Falls, fractures, and hip pads." *Curr Osteoporos Rep*. 2004 Dec;2(4):131-7. (Review)

Sinaki M, et al. "Balance disorder and increased risk of falls in osteoporosis and kyphosis: significance of kyphotic posture and muscle strength." *Osteoporos Int*. 2005 Aug;16(8):1004-10.

Sinaki M. "The role of physical activity in bone health: a new hypothesis to reduce risk of vertebral fracture." *Phys Med Rehabil Clin N Am*. 2007 Aug;18(3):593-608, xi-xii. (Review)

Slemenda CW, et. al. "Role of physical activity in the development of skeletal mass in children." *J Bone Min Res* 1991;6:1227-1233.

Smith EL, et. al., "Effects of inactivity and exercise on bone." *The Physician and Sports Medicine* 1987;15:91-100.

Smith EL, "Exercise for prevention of osteoporosis: A review." *The Phys and Sports Med* 1982; 10(3):72-82.

Smith EL, Gilligan C, "Mechanical forces and bone (a review)." Ed. by WA Peck, *Bone Min Res* 1989:139-173.

Smith EL, et. al., "Deterring bone loss by exercise intervention in premenopausal and post-menopausal women." *Calcification Tissue International* 1989;44:312-321.

Smith EL, Raab DM. Osteoporosis and physical activity. Acta med Scand Suppl. 1986;711:149-56.

Smith EL & Gilligan C. "Physical activity effects on bone metabolism." *Calcified Tissue International.* 1991; 49(Suppl.), S50-4.

Smith L, "Bone Concerns." *Women and Exercise: Physiology and Sports Medicine.* Ed. By MM Shangold and G Mirkin. Philadelphia:FA Davis and Co., 1988.

Snow-Harter CM, "Bone Health and prevention of osteoporosis in active and athletic women." *Clin Sports Med* 1994 Apr;13(2):389-404.

Swanenburg J, et al. "Effects of exercise and nutrition on postural balance and risk of falling in elderly people with decreased bone mineral density: randomized controlled trial pilot study." *Clin Rehabil.* 2007 Jun;21(6):523-34.

Taaffe DR, Robinson TL, Snow CM, Marcus R. High-impact exercise promotes bone gain in well-trained female athletes. J Bone Miner Res. 1997 Feb;12(2):255-60.

Tosi LL, et al. "The American Orthopaedic Association's "own the bone" initiative to prevent secondary fractures." *J Bone Joint Surg Am.* 2008 Jan;90(1):163-73.

Turner CH, & Robling AG. "Exercises for improving bone strength." Br J Sports Med. 2005 Apr;39(4):188-9.
US Dept. of Health and Human Services (HHS). "Bone Heath and Osteoporosis-A Report of the Surgeon General." Public Health Services, Office of the Surgeon General, Rockville, MD; 2004.

Vaillant J, et al. "Balance, aging, and osteoporosis: effects of cognitive exercises combined with physiotherapy." *Joint Bone Spine.* 2006 Jul;73(4):414-8.

Velez NF, et al. "The effect of moderate impact exercise on skeletal integrity in master athletes." *Osteoporos Int.* 2008 Mar 20.

Wainwright SA, et al. "Study of Osteoporotic Fractures Research Group. Hip fracture in women without osteoporosis." *J Clin Endocrinol Metab.* 2005 May;90(5):2787-93.

Wayne PM, et al. "The effects of Tai Chi on bone mineral density in postmenopausal women: a systematic review." *Arch Phys Med Rehabil.* 2007 May;88(5):673-80. (Review)

Whalen RT, et. al., "Influence of physical activity on the regulation of bone density." *J of Biomechanics* 1998;21:825-837.

Wilkins CH, Birge SJ. "Prevention of osteoporotic fractures in the elderly." *Am J Med.* 2005 Nov;118(11):1190-5. (Review)

Winters KM, Snow CM. "Detraining reverses positive effects of exercise on the musculoskeletal system in premenopausal women." *J Bone Miner Res.* 2000 Dec;15(12):2495-503.

Winters-Stone KM, Snow CM. "Musculoskeletal response to exercise is greatest in women with low initial values." *Med Sci Sports Exerc*. 2003 Oct;35(10):1691-6.

Winters-Stone KM, Snow CM. "Site-specific response of bone to exercise in premenopausal women." *Bone.* 2006 Dec;39(6):1203-9.

Wolf SL, et al. "The effect of Tai Chi Quan and Computerized Balance Training on Postural Stability in Older Subjects." *Physical Therapy* 1997;77(4):371-384.

Wolf SL, Barnhart HX, Kutner NG, McNeely E, Coogler C, Xu T; Atlanta FICSIT Group. Selected as the best paper in the 1990s: Reducing frailty and falls in older persons: an investigation of tai chi and computerized balance training. J Am Geriatr Soc. 2003 Dec;51(12):1794-803.

Wright JD, Wang CY, Kennedy-Stevenson J, Ervin RB. Dietary intakes of ten key nutrients for public health, United States: 1999-2000. Adv Data 2003 Apr 17;(334):104. Hyattsville Maryland: National Center on Health Statistics. 2003.

Zehnacker CH, Bemis-Dougherty A. "Effect of weighted exercises on bone mineral density in post menopausal women. A systematic review." *J Geriatr Phys Ther.* 2007;30(2):79-88. (Review)

About the Author

SHERRI R. BETZ, PT is a 1991 graduate of the Louisiana State University Medical Center School of Physical Therapy. Sherri actually began her career as a national gymnastics competitor and as a group fitness instructor and personal trainer for Nautilus Fitness Centers in the 1980's. Inspired by the work of a physical therapist in one of the clubs where she trained, Sherri began to pursue a degree in physical therapy.

Her love of movement education has been integrated into her physical therapy practice at a rehabilitative level and at a fitness level. Utilization of Pilates-based methods and Gyrotonic® with a specialty in the treatment of the pelvic girdle and manual therapy of the spine are integral in her practice as a Physical Therapist.

As Director of Pilates-Based Programs for Western Athletic Clubs at Courtside Club in Los Gatos, CA, she continues to conduct classes, seminars and instructor training programs. Sherri has developed programs for the San Jose Sharks professional hockey team, nationally ranked pairs and singles figure skaters, and elite-level gymnasts in their rehabilitation and in development of their Pilates-based training programs.

As a member of the American Physical Therapy Association's Women's Health Section, and Director of Physical Therapy and Exercise Programs for Heart to Hearts, Inc.: Empowering Women Through Education in Lawrenceville, NJ, she has developed Women's and Corporate Wellness Programs for ergonomics, exercise, osteoporosis, nutrition, use of herbs, menopause education, hormone replacement therapy, cancer prevention, and stress reduction.

Sherri has been a principal educator and examiner for **Polestar Education** since 1999 and is certified in Gyrotonic®, and GyrokinesisTM. She has developed an advanced program in Osteoporosis Management for Polestar Education. Extensive research on the treatment and prevention of Osteoporosis and Osteoarthritis led to the development of *The Osteoporosis Exercise Book: Building Better Bones*, and the following DVD's: *Pilates for Osteoporosis, Prenatal Pilates, Dealing with Acute Low Back Pain*, and newest DVD, *Pilates for Seniors*.

Sherri is currently working on a new edition *of The Osteoporosis Exercise Book* with integration of Pilates and Physical Therapy principles and exercise modifications for those at risk for fracture. Sherri has served on the Board of Directors for the Pilates Method Alliance since 2003. She became **PMA Pilates Gold Certified** in 2005 and served on the PMA Pilates Certification Exam National Panel to improve the quality, safety and standards of Pilates Instruction. Sherri also is enjoying her role working with some incredible people on the Professional Education Committee for FORE (Foundation for Osteoporosis Research and Education).

Sherri's motto's and life goals are: 1)To inspire and assist people in movement without pain 2)To change faulty habitual patterns of movement and create new healthy patterns of movement   3)Exercise should be fun!   4)Aging does not mean decline!

Sherri lives with her husband, Jugdeep Aggarwal and their beloved Yorkshire Terrier, "Cali", in Santa Cruz, CA and owns TheraPilates®, a physical therapy, Pilates and Gyrotonic® Clinic.

101

To inquire about, schedule or enroll in upcoming courses or to purchase books or videos you can find Sherri on the web at:

www.TheraPilates.com   Email: Sherri@TheraPilates.com   Phone: 831-476-3100
www.Amazon.com
www.BalancedBody.com
www.PolestarPilates.com

For more information about osteoporosis and updates go to:

www.FORE.org
www.NOF.org
www.osteofound.org

If you have a question about osteoporosis or exercise, ask it on our Blog at www.TheraPilates.com/blog.

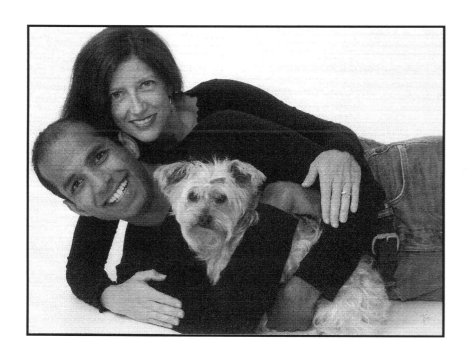

102

NOTES:

NOTES:

NOTES:

NOTES:

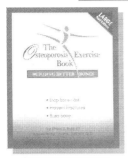

The Osteoporosis Exercise Book: Building Better Bones, 2ⁿᵈ Ed. was written to help you incorporate safe mat exercises into your bone-building program. The exercises will help you build bone density of the spine and hip, improve posture and balance, and increase flexibility and mobility from beginner to the advanced level exerciser. You will also learn how to avoid movements that increase the risk of fracture. Includes photos, nutritional recommendations, fracture prevention and some of the latest research findings on Osteoporosis. Over 100 photos, 104 pages.   **By Sherri R. Betz, PT**

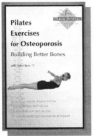

Pilates Exercises for Osteoporosis DVD was designed by physical therapist, Sherri Betz to help you incorporate safe Pilates exercises into your bone building program. Many Pilates exercises can be unsafe and contraindicated for those with low bone density. By modifying the wonderful exercises of Joseph Pilates and incorporating sound physical therapy principles, you will learn the best exercises to build the bones of the most vulnerable areas of the hip and spinal vertebrae.   *PAL & NTSC*   **57 minutes**

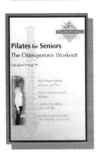

Pilates for Seniors: The Osteoporosis Workout DVD was developed for Seniors or those who have difficulty getting up and down from the floor for exercises. Explanation of anatomy, proper breathing, spine positioning and deep abdominal contraction precedes the workout. All exercises done in seated or standing position. Includes instructions for safely getting down to and up off the floor without risk for fracture and a few exercises suggestions for exercises that can be done in bed.   *PAL & NTSC* By Sherri Betz, PT   **64 minutes**

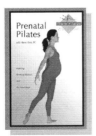

Prenatal Pilates DVD was developed by Sherri Betz, Physical Therapist, Polestar Pilates Educator and Women's Health Specialist, using guidelines from the American College of Obstetrics and Gynecology. Introduction to proper breathing, spine alignment, transversus abdominus contractions, diastasis recti, and abdominal anatomy followed by a prenatal mat class. All 3 Trimester modifications are demonstrated with precautions and contraindications for a safe workout.   *PAL & NTSC*   **1 Hour 22 minutes**

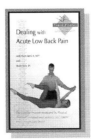

Dealing with Acute Low Back Pain DVD was developed to enhance the progress and effectiveness of a physical therapy program for patients with Acute Low Back Injuries. Due to shrinking reimbursement by health insurances, physical therapists are often very limited in the time they have with patients and often the treatment programs cannot be completed, restoring patients to full pre-injury status. Included are several principles and basic skills that most patients with spine or lumbo-pelvic injuries should learn prevent further injury and allow healing to occur as rapidly as possible.   *PAL & NTSC*   **55 minutes**

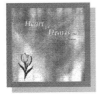

The Heart to Hearts, Inc. Meditation CD was designed to give you an experience of relaxation and meditation. The proceeds of this CD go to support the Heart to Hearts Women's Wellness Program, a Non-Profit Foundation whose goal is to "Empower Women through Education". Narrated by Sherri Betz, PT. Music by Kevin Halliez. **45 minutes**

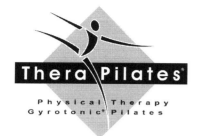

1. PILATES FOR OSTEOPOROSIS DVD
2. PILATES FOR SENIORS DVD
3. DEALING WITH ACUTE LOW BACK PAIN DVD
4. PRENATAL PILATES DVD
5. THE OSTEOPOROSIS EXERCISE BOOK, 2nd Ed.
6. THE HEART TO HEARTS MEDITATION CD

Name:_____

Organization:_____

Shipping Address:_____

City:_____ State:_____ Zip/Postal Code:_____

Phone Home:_____ Work:_____

Cell Phone:_____ Fax:_____

Email Address:_____

Number of Osteoporosis DVD's: _____ x 24.95 = Subtotal: _____

Number of Senior Videos: _____ x 24.95 = Subtotal: _____

Number of Low Back Pain DVD's: _____ x 24.95 = Subtotal: _____

Number of Prenatal Pilates DVD's:_____ x 24.95 = Subtotal: _____

Number of Osteoporosis Books : _____ x 19.95 = Subtotal: _____

Number of Meditation CD's: _____ x 14.95 = Subtotal: _____

8.5% Tax (CA) : _____

Shipping & Handling- $6 for 1-2 items $10 for 3 or more items: $_____

TOTAL: $_____

VISA or MASTERCARD #_____ - _____ - _____ - _____

Expiration Date_____ **Name on Card**_____

Billing Address _____

City_____ **State**_____ **Zip Code**_____

Or send Check or Money Order Payable to:
Call Toll Free 888-229-5334

TheraPilates
920-A 41st Avenue
Santa Cruz, CA 95062